AGING MEDICINE

Robert J. Pignolo, MD, PhD; Mary Ann Forciea, MD;
Jerry C. Johnson, MD, Series Editors

For other titles published in this series, go to
www.springer.com/series/7622

F. Michael Gloth, III
Editor

Handbook of Pain Relief in Older Adults

An Evidence-Based Approach

Second Edition

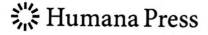 Humana Press

Editor
F. Michael Gloth, III, MD
Division of Geriatric Medicine and Gerontology
Johns Hopkins University School of Medicine
Baltimore, MD
USA
fgloth1@jhmi.edu

ISBN 978-1-60761-617-7   e-ISBN 978-1-60761-618-4
DOI 10.1007/978-1-60761-618-4
Springer New York Dordrecht Heidelberg London

Printed on acid-free paper

Humana Press is part of Springer Science+Business Media (www.springer.com)

Preface

Since publication of the first edition of the *Handbook of Pain Relief in Older Adults*, much has changed. Drugs once felt to be safer for older adults have been removed from the market for safety reasons. New guidelines on the management of persistent pain in older adults have been published, and, of course, new drugs and interventions have been developed. This second edition of the *Handbook of Pain Relief in Older Adults* once again provides useful information from some of the leading experts in the pain field from around the USA. Again there has been a reliance on evidence that has been gleaned from the scientific literature or from the research of the respective authors. Where data are inadequate to form definitive conclusions, the text uses the best evidence available and expert opinion, assimilating the knowledge from the rich clinical experience available to the authors along with the available clinical study experience. Wherever evidence is lacking, an effort has been made to express that.

The pain field is changing so rapidly, with so many new discoveries, that one must accept the fact that by the time this textbook is published, there may be new interventions available. However, the guiding principles of the *Handbook of Pain Relief in Older Adults* will persist long after the pages on the text are worn and frayed.

Intrinsic to this book is the concept that pain can always be treated and that treatment will be most effective when the etiology for the pain is understood. In addition to the treatment for pain, we cannot overlook the importance of interventions to prevent or minimize the onset of pain. Pain assessment must be a primary focus of any care plan aimed at managing pain.

Pain does not discriminate. People from any setting can experience pain. Efforts to assess and treat pain should be directed to the individual while recognizing that not all assessment tools or interventions will be as useful in all populations. Whatever instrument is used should be selected based on standardized testing in populations similar to individuals being evaluated.

Medications and medical science are only a small part of the equation for controlling pain in our society. The reader of this second edition of the *Handbook of Pain Relief in Older Adults* should learn new holistic strategies for helping to provide comfort and dignity for those who suffer from pain.

Finally, it is important to publicly acknowledge and thank those who contributed so much to allowing this book to become a reality. Greatly appreciated are the efforts of Mr. Richard Lansing, who recognized the need for this second edition and who encouraged us to move forward on this project. In addition, all the contributing authors, without whom this text would have never become a reality, also have my unending gratitude. They have truly raised the bar in producing such a quality product. Thanks also go to my loving family. Such unending support is crucial for such a work to come to fruition. My wife, Maybian, must be singled out for she is one of the greatest blessings in my life. Also, thanks to my loving daughters, Anna, Kate, Jane, and Molly, who bring such joy to the world and provide much needed relief and support in so many ways. Finally, and most importantly, praise is due to God. *Nisi Dominus, frustra.*

Maryland, 2010

Contents

Contributors

Richard A. Black, PT, DPT, MS, GCS
Corporate Rehabilitation Consultant, HCR ManorCare,
333 N. Summit Street, Toledo, OH 43606
rblack@hcr-manorcare.com

Micke Brown, BSN, RN
Communication Director, American Pain Foundation,
mbrown@painfoundation.org

Susan L. Charette, MD
Assistant Clinical Professor, UCLA Division of Geriatrics,
200 UCLA Medical Plaza, Suite 420, Los Angeles, CA 90095, USA
scharette@mednet.ucla.edu

Amanda Crowe, MA, MPH
President and Founder, Impact Health Communications, LLC
amandacrowe@hotmail.com

Bruce A. Ferrell, MD
Associate Professor, UCLA Division of Geriatrics,
10945 Le Conte Avenue, Suite 2339, Los Angeles, CA 90095, USA
BFerrell@mednet.ucla.edu

F. Michael Gloth, III, MD
Associate Professor, Division of Geriatric Medicine and Gerontology,
Johns Hopkins University School of Medicine, Baltimore, MD, USA
fgloth1@jhmi.edu

Mark J. Gloth, DO
Corporate Medical Director, HCR ManorCare, 333 N. Summit Street,
Toledo, Ohio 43699-0086
magloth@hcr-manorcare.com

Frederick W. Luthardt, MA
Johns Hopkins University School of Medicine, 550 N. Broadway,
Suite 301, Baltimore, MD 21205, USA

Mary Lynn McPherson, Pharm.D., BCPS, CPE
Professor and Vice Chair, Department of Pharmacy Practice and Science,
University of Maryland School of Pharmacy, 20 N. Pine Street, Room 405,
Baltimore, Maryland 21201, USA
mmcphers@rx.umaryland.edu

Thomas Mulligan, MD
Medical Director, Senior Services, St. Bernards Health Care,
Jonesboro, AR, USA
tmulligan@sbrmc.org

Maneesh C. Sharma, MD
Johns Hopkins University School of Medicine, 550 N. Broadway,
Suite 301, Baltimore, MD 21205, USA

Cristina Rosca Sichitiu, MD
Medical Director Hospice, St. Bernards Health Care,
225 E. Jackson Avenue, Jonesboro, AR 72401-3119, USA

Peter S. Staats, MD, MBA
Adjunct Associate Professor, Department of Anesthesiology
and Critical Care Medicine, Department of Oncology at Johns Hopkins,
University School of Medicine in Baltimore, Maryland,
Premier Pain Management, Shrewsbury, NJ, USA
pstaats@jhmi.edu

Tanya J. Uritsky, Pharm.D.
Hospital of the University of Pennsylvania, Philadelphia, PA, USA

Kulbir S. Walia, MD
Premier Pain Centers, 160 Avenue at the Common Shrewsbury, NJ, USA

Chapter 1
Introduction

F. Michael Gloth, III

The greater the ignorance, the greater the dogmatism.

Sir William Osler

For many who have entered the field of health care, one major factor was the desire to help others through the relief of suffering. Pain is often an element of suffering. The International Association for the Study of Pain defines "pain" as "an unpleasant sensory and emotional experience associated with actual or potential tissue damage, or described in terms of such damage or both" [1]. There are many subclasses that have been proposed, e.g., acute, chronic, or persistent. There have also been suggestions of describing pain with such terms as visceral, neuropathic, nociceptive, psychological, musculoskeletal, psychosomatic, etc. Some of these terms are used in this text as well. Such terms are useful only if they help to describe the etiology of the pain or discomfort, and, thus, facilitate treatment. Their usefulness is somewhat dependent upon others recognizing their definitions as well. If terminology begins to hinder communication, one must question its utility overall.

Another area of frequent discussion in the literature involves the terms "opioids" and "opiates." "Opioid" is defined as, "any synthetic narcotic that has opiate-like activities but is not derived from opium" [2]. Therefore, drugs like fentanyl, hydrocodone, and oxycodone are classified as opioids, while morphine would be an opiate. For the sake of simplicity, this second edition of the *Handbook of Pain Relief in Older Adults* retains the convention of using the term "opioid" for both. Because of the negative connotation of the term "narcotic" in association with illicit drug use, that term will be avoided throughout this text, and it is recommended that it not be used in clinical practice. Regardless of the terminology chosen, pain of longer duration and/or of an unremitting nature has the potential to wear an individual down in every conceivable way, including emotionally, physically, spiritually, and socially.

F.M. Gloth, III (✉)
Division of Geriatric Medicine and Gerontology, Johns Hopkins University
School of Medicine, Baltimore, MD, USA
e-mail: fgloth1@jhmi.edu

F.M. Gloth, III (ed.), *Handbook of Pain Relief in Older Adults: An Evidence-Based Approach*, Aging Medicine, DOI 10.1007/978-1-60761-618-4_1,
© Springer Science+Business Media, LLC 2011

1

Regrettably, data indicate that all too often, health-care professionals fail in resolving pain, one of the clearest factors associated with suffering [3, 4]. This is especially true when the person in pain is a senior. Simply knowing that pain exists is not sufficient. There must also be proper assessment, and, of course, proper intervention. Even this approach is incomplete. To be complete, there must also be attention to prevention of pain as well. This edition of the *Handbook of Pain Relief in Older Adults* was written to provide an updated and comprehensive approach to relieving suffering in older adults through relief of their pain.

Through an evidence-based approach the contributors provide information on the scope of the problem, insight into assessing pain status, and practical guidance for treatment. Somewhat unique is the discussion of steps to prevent pain in seniors. It is not adequate for us to act after pain has developed. Rather, efforts must be made to prevent, or at least minimize, pain when circumstances that are likely to produce this devil are identifiable. This text has addressed many of the standard issues in pain management. Most importantly, however, is the effort to address other aspects of pain. Once again, Dr. Mulligan's team, provide insight into the role of spirituality as an adjunct to pain management. The internet and computerized patient records is now commonly used to foster improved care and once again is addressed in the text. New in this edition is a chapter by Micke Brown, BSN, RN (Executive Director of the American Pain Foundation) and Amanda Crowe, MA, MPH (Health Communication Consultant for the American Pain Foundation and founder of IMPACT Health Communications, LLC) on resources that are available for patients with pain and for the professionals who work with them.

The recognition that direct efforts targeted at pain management comprise only part of the approach to pain resolution, has led to a repeat effort in this edition to examine other indirect factors, such as availability of resources and excessive regulation, which should be recognized as paramount in achieving successful pain management. For the older adult, where Medicare is only one of the regulatory agencies overseeing care, the process can be more challenging, as well-intended regulations sometimes are responsible for inflicting more pain than they resolve. The impact of legislation and public policy must also be appreciated in an even broader sense with seniors. As this edition goes to press, ineluctable Congressional inaction, Federal Code, and regulatory actions from the Drug Enforcement Agency in long-term care have stifled efforts to make opioids available to seniors who need them in the nursing home setting. As a result, some of the most frail and vulnerable citizens of the country are made to suffer needlessly.

Other strategies must also recognize patient autonomy. Patients in pain will independently struggle for more information and, hopefully, more relief. The chapter devoted to internet resources and electronic medical records should prove valuable for clinicians as well as patient. The chapter by Browne and Crowe should prove to be most valuable to those looking for additional resources. Helping patients and caregivers to advocate for adequate pain management is also addressed in the latter chapters. It is recognized that all clinicians can't be experts. It is important for individuals to recognize that if adequate pain relief is not obtained, there are other options, which may include other physicians. Hopefully, such referrals can be directed by primary-care clinicians with appropriate understanding and humility to make those referrals early and often.

The politics of pain management are addressed as well as the impact of the media. The politics of pain are by no means confined to legislation debated on Capitol Hill nor at state capitols throughout the country (or in any other country for that matter). The politics of pain ensnares even the most ardent pain management advocate and the discussion of this issue should help in the battle to provide better pain relief everywhere. How this plays out in the media is not always under control. At times media resources not only contribute to poor pain management, but as later chapters illustrate may actually exacerbate pain, albeit indirectly. As an author, I recognize another media contribution herein, yet am optimistic that there are still some opportunities for positive and, dare I speculate, even responsible contributions. It is my fervent hope that the *Handbook of Pain Relief in Older Adults* 2nd Edition achieves such a level of contribution to the literature.

Finally, there is a chapter for the future. This chapter provides suggestions to accomplish pain relief over a broad spectrum. Suggestions target individuals as well as large-scale endeavors. The challenge of pain relief for the rapidly increasing body of seniors must be addressed now if we are to have any hope of living in comfort in the days and years ahead. It is a challenge for all of us. This book is only one of many sparks that must be lit to create a blazing effort to eliminate the omnipresent shadow of pain throughout the world. To move forward in the fiery and passionate advocacy of pain relief, we must recognize that one of the worst marriages is that of ignorance and arrogance; and, thus, it will be important to maintain an open perspective and to fill the knowledge void with as much factual information as possible. With steadfast efforts from all who read these words, all of us can look forward to a much brighter future as we meet the pain relief challenge.

References

1. Merskey H, Bogduk N, editors. Classification of chronic pain, 2nd ed. Seattle: IASP; 1994. p. xi–xv
2. The Free dictionary. http://medical-dictionary.thefreedictionary.com/opioid. Accessed 11 May 2010.
3. Gloth FM III. Pain management in older adults: prevention and treatment. J Am Geriatr Soc. 2001;49:188–99.
4. CDC. Prevalence of disabilities and associated health conditions among adults – United States, 1999. MMWR Morb Mortal Wkly Rep. 2001;50:120–5.

Chapter 2
Pain, Pain Everywhere...Almost

F. Michael Gloth, III

There was a faith healer from Deal
Who said, "Although pain isn't real
When I sit on a pin
And it punctures my skin
I dislike what I fancy I feel."

English Limerick

Reports on the prevalence of pain in our society are staggering. This is particularly true for seniors [1]. Data indicate that half of the people over the age of 65 are not functioning at their optimal level because of interference from pain [2–4]. In 1997, a telephone survey was reported as indicating that >50% of older adults had taken prescriptions of pain medication beyond a 6-month period and that 45% had seen at least three physicians for pain, in the prior 5 years [5]. For certain populations, the numbers are even more disconcerting. For example, in a nursing-home environment, estimates are that anywhere from half to 80% of residents have pain, with analgesics being used in 40–50% of residents [6–9]. Further analysis indicates that almost a quarter of patients with daily pain did not receive any analgesics [10]. Additionally, long-term care data indicate that over 40% of patients, who were known to have pain at an initial assessment, had worsening or severe pain at the time of the second assessment 2–6 months later [11]. Many of these seniors, including those with diseases recognized to have a strong association with pain, such as cancer, are inadequately or not treated at all with analgesics [12, 13]. Even dying patients can be expected to suffer persistent severe pain in the long-term care setting, at rates exceeding 40% [11].

Pain exacts a terrible toll on our society as well as the individuals who directly suffer from pain. In 2005, the White House Conference on Aging identified pain management among the top 50 priorities in the next decade (Resolution 21: Improve The Health and Quality of Life of Older Americans Through Disease Management and Chronic Care Coordination and Resolution 34: Reduce Healthcare Disparities

F.M. Gloth, III (✉)
Division of Geriatric Medicine and Gerontology, Johns Hopkins University School of Medicine, Baltimore, MD, USA
e-mail: fgloth1@jhmi.edu

F.M. Gloth, III (ed.), *Handbook of Pain Relief in Older Adults: An Evidence-Based Approach*, Aging Medicine, DOI 10.1007/978-1-60761-618-4_2,
© Springer Science+Business Media, LLC 2011

Among Minorities by Developing Strategies to Prevent Disease, Promote Health, and Deliver Appropriate Care and Wellness from http://www.whcoa.gov). Patients with pain are more likely to have a host of other complications associated with pain [10, 14]. The overwhelming majority (98% in one study) of patients who finally do get to a pain center for chronic pain have developed a psychiatric diagnosis as well [15]. In veterans, estimates are that 70% have some pain-related disability [16]. These effects have a direct negative impact on physical and cognitive functioning in suffering patients, and, indirectly, spouses, family, and other caregivers suffer as well [17, 18].

Pain is not a normal part of aging, and it may present differently in different cultures, populations, or settings. Perhaps the most common differences have been reported between males and females. Women may experience pain differently than men. For example, women may report higher levels of pain, but they also are more likely to have chronic conditions associated with pain [19]. Whether or not there are true sex differences in pain perception or pain reporting, however, remains open for discussion [20].

- One is likely to encounter a greater prevalence of painful syndromes in the older adult compared to younger counterparts [21–23]. For example, neuropathic pain is quite common. In older adults, diabetes and Varicella (the virus that causes chicken pox and shingles) are common causes of neuropathic or nerve pain. Herpes zoster or shingles attacks over half a million Americans each year. Almost one in 12 report pain at 1 month, and about half of those still have pain at 1 year. This postherpetic neuralgia with prolonged pain is more common among people older than 60 years of age [24]. Over half of patients with slowly progressive neuromuscular disease report moderate to very severe pain [25]. Arthritis alone affects well over 20 million Americans with an increase to 40 million expected by 2020 [26]. Twenty-nine percent of Medicare patients in nursing homes with a fracture in the prior 6 months suffer with daily pain [27].

Terminology Issues

Pain may be even more prevalent than some figures indicate. The term "pain" may be avoided, with preference for "discomfort," "ache," "hurt," "crick," or a plethora of other terms that make up the pain vernacular. For this reason, inclusion of other terms and colloquialisms germane to the population being evaluated is necessary.

The medical community also has a variety of terms that need to be recognized and understood for adequate communication regarding pain. The International Association for the Study of Pain developed a Subcommittee on Taxonomy in the late 1980s to define and clarify many of the medical terms used in the field [28]. Some of the more common terms and definitions appear below:

Allodynia – pain due to a stimulus which does not normally provoke pain.
Analgesia – absence of pain in response to stimulation which would normally
    be painful.

Anesthesia dolorosa – pain in an area or region which is anesthetic.

Causalgia (complex regional pain syndrome) – a syndrome of sustained burning pain, allodynia, and hyperpathia after traumatic nerve lesion, often combined with vasomotor dysfunction.

Central pain – pain associated with the central nervous system.

Dysesthesia – an unpleasant abnormal sensation, whether spontaneous or evoked.

Hyperesthesia – increased sensitivity to stimulation, excluding the special senses.

Hyperalgesia – an increased response to a stimulus, which is normally painful

Hyperpathia – a painful syndrome, characterized by increased reaction to a stimulus, especially a repetitive stimulus, as well as increased threshold.

Hypoesthesia – decreased sensitivity to stimulation, excluding the special senses.

Hypoalgesia – diminished pain in response to normally painful stimulus.

Neuralgia – pain in the distribution of a nerve or nerves.

Neuritis – inflammation of a nerve or nerves.

Neuropathy – a disturbance of function or pathological change in a nerve; in one nerve, mononeuropathy; in several nerves, mononeuropathy multiplex; if diffuse and bilateral, polyneuropathy.

Nociceptor – a receptor preferentially sensitive to a noxious stimulus or to a stimulus which would become noxious if prolonged.

Noxious stimulus – a stimulus which is damaging, or potentially so, to normal tissues.

Pain threshold – the least experience of pain which a subject can recognize.

Pain tolerance level – the greatest level of pain which a subject is prepared to tolerate.

Paresthesia – an abnormal sensation, whether spontaneous or evoked.

Reasons for Poor Pain Control in Seniors

Despite such high prevalence of pain and painful syndromes in older adults, there have been relatively few studies in older populations with pain [29]. Studies have indicated that <1% of the thousands of papers published on pain focus on the aging society [30]. This lack of research may explain part of the failure to provide adequate pain relief to seniors. A variety of other factors also seem to contribute to the dismal performance of the health-care profession in providing substantial pain relief to older adults in pain.

The reasons cited for lagging performance at the clinician level include inadequate training, lack of effort to obtain appropriate assessment (including the use of formal assessment instruments), and reluctance to prescribe opioids [31, 32]. The lack of knowledge due to inadequate training may foster some of the other reasons mentioned [33]. Ironically, health-care professionals acknowledge receiving inadequate instruction on pain management during medical school and residency training, which may explain the inadequate prescribing of analgesics [34, 35]. Oftentimes, what has been learned seems to be incorrect, as an exaggerated opinion about the effects of opioids with regard to addiction, tolerance, respiratory depression, and sedation is expressed by many health care professionals [30, 36].

Patients have also been responsible for some of the lack of success in managing pain. Fears associated with taking opioids and a reluctance to report pain have created additional obstacles in the efforts to overcome pain [30]. Most of the concerns are not based in fact. Addiction rarely occurs in anyone taking opioids for pain. In reality, addiction risk with opioids is low (<0.1%) when analgesics are used for acute pain in patients who are not substance abusers [37]. Even chronic use of morphine rarely leads to addiction when used to control pain [38]. Multiple studies have shown that people taking chronic opioids function similarly to those with no medications [39]. Even driving ability with long-term morphine use for analgesia in cancer patients was not substantially different than those without such medication [40]. Reflecting these facts, the American Geriatrics Society released new guidelines on Persistent Pain in Older Persons: Pharmacological Management of Persistent Pain in Older Persons in May of 2009, advocating the use of opioids in persistent pain situations that did not respond to nonopioid medications [41].

In a survey of nursing-home residents, some other factors that may impair the inclination of residents to report pain were identified [42]. In this survey, residents expressed the opinion that the staff lacked the time to adequately assess and treat pain. There was also a sentiment that if pain did not impair function, then treatment of persistent pain was unnecessary. Also expressed was the belief that it was not reasonable to complain of pain if there was not a physical deformity or well-defined pathology. Oftentimes, there is a false impression that pain is a normal consequence of getting older and that once chronic pain develops, there is little potential of responding to treatment.

Additional barriers to adequate pain control exist. These encompass not only those from the health-care professional and the patient but also various institutional barriers [43–45]. Additional factors based on the source include:

Senior patients – Beliefs that pain cannot be avoided and should simply be tolerated, reluctance to discuss pain symptoms unless explicitly asked, misinformation about opioids (e.g., addiction potential or likelihood and degree of side effects), lack of display of typical signs and symptoms or display to a lesser degree than younger patients, cognitive or sensory impairment that limits ability to report pain, and biases may hinder patients from reporting pain, coexisting illnesses (especially depression) may reduce a patient's ability to interpret or report pain, medications may modify responses to pain, and pain may be misconstrued to be an inevitable consequence of aging, a punishment for past actions, or something that cannot or will not be treated or will incur the ill feelings of care providers if a complaint is registered.

Health professionals – Lack of training or skill at using assessment techniques and screening instruments, inadequate knowledge about opioids, overestimation of rates of addiction and respiratory depression, belief that pain is a normal part of aging, provision of care by individuals without formal pain management training, disbelief of a patient's report of pain, reluctance to refer for consultation in a timely fashion, or belief that sleep following administration of pain medication is due to an adverse event from the medication rather than a normal response of an exhausted person who has finally achieved a level of comfort.

Institutional or system – High turnover of staff limits the experience in using pain assessment techniques. Lack of a systematic approach to screening and prevention, inherent inefficiencies in the use of ancillary health-care personnel, lack of individual accountability within the system, poorly functioning care teams, poor leadership and commitment to pain management at a management level, and excessive regulations (especially in long-term care) may result in failure to give priority to recognition, assessment, and treatment of pain. Extensive documentation requirement (particularly with opioids) may deter health-care professionals from appropriately prescribing effective treatments. This may also impose time constraints, which may impede physicians from focusing adequately on pain control. Other factors such as inadequate reimbursement and financial incentives for pain management efforts, negative reinforcement in training programs for attending to pain while being rewarded for less important and more detailed interventions such as daily laboratory blood testing of metabolic profiles, lack of training for pain management skills, lack of recognition and interaction among various medical disciplines (and even among different pain groups), limited access to diagnostic or therapeutic facilities or experts, inadequate pharmacy services (including insufficient stocking of medications for pain, like opioids), insufficient staffing for proper pain assessment and interventions, inflexible access to medications based on formulary selections, and other restrictive policies and procedures may also contribute to failure in treatment of pain (Table 2.1).

There are other areas for improvement. Despite the fact that two third of people who consider a nursing home their place of residence will die there, few of them will ever be enrolled in hospice [46]. In a later chapter on "suggestions for change," the roles of patient, health-care professional, and systems are addressed as they pertain to improved hospice referral to optimize end-of-life pain care.

Treatment and Recurrent Pain

One of the challenges for clinicians working in the field of pain management is the modification of behavior that follows adequate treatment of pain. Once pain relief is achieved, a patient is very likely to enter a cycle not generally discussed (Fig. 2.1). Once pain is controlled, an individual usually becomes more functional and then more active. This can lead to irritation of the area that previously caused pain. Such irritation can lead to increased inflammation and consequently, a recurrence of pain. Thus, successful pain control is perceived as short-lived, and this cyclical process

Table 2.1 Obstacles to good pain management in older adults

Patient-related	Health professional-related	System-related
• Fears of addiction with opioids· Reluctance to report pain	• Inadequate training· Lack of assessment	• Insufficient research
• Lack of confidence in response to reporting pain	• Misinformation about addiction with opioids	• High staff turnover with new staff unfamiliar with assessment and treatment techniques
• False belief that without defined pathology or loss of function treatment is not necessary	• Exaggerated risk of respiratory depression with opioids	• Lack of individual accountability within the system
• False belief that pain is a normal part of aging	• Misinterpretation of sedation with opioids	• Poor oversight and functioning of care teams
• Fear of being labeled a "bad" patient	• Ignorance of development of tolerance to nausea etc. with opioids	• Inadequate administrative support for pain management efforts
• Misconception that chronic pain is not amenable to therapy	• Lack of time/priority for diagnosis and treatment	• Lack of trained leadership
• Lack of typical signs and symptoms compared to younger patients	• False belief that pain is a normal part of aging	• Excessive regulation
• Comorbid conditions or medications may affect the ability to report pain	• Disbelief in patient's report of pain	• Overly burdensome documentation requirements
	• Misinterpreting sleep as medication-induced somnolence	• Inadequate reimbursement for pain management
	• Reluctance to refer	• Insufficient access to resources and training

Pain-Treatment-Pain Pentagon©

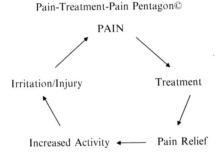

Fig. 2.1 The Pain Pentagon represents a cycle of pain, treatment, improved function and activity, producing further local irritation or remote injury, resulting in new or recurrent pain. This illustrates the risk of reinjury and the potential impact of increased activity accompanying successful pain intervention, which paradoxically may strain deconditioned areas of the body after long periods of rest due to prior underlying discomfort. Used with permission. © 2003 F. Michael Gloth, III, M.D. Used with permission

makes good pain control more challenging. This sequence of events should be recognized so that adequate counseling can take place to prevent such a cycle of pain.

It also should be recognized that prolonged pain could lead to disuse atrophy. Again, the resolution of pain may lead to further activity. In this setting, the lack of muscular balance may be associated with misalignment of the spine or increased trauma on insufficiently supported joints. Consequently, injury and pain can result (Fig. 2.1).

More Regulation Not the Answer

While there has been some progress, it has been very slow and minimal, at best, with pain rates still far too high [47]. Oftentimes, bureaucrats, health policy makers, and legislators try to resolve issues with even more regulations or laws. Additional regulation does not seem to be the answer, and neither will more government oversight prove to be beneficial. While the intent of additional regulation is often admirable, it is important to assess the impact of regulations. In a study of the impact of the Omnibus Budget Reconciliation Act of 1987 on the tangible measurement of pressure sores in nursing-home residents, Coleman et al. showed no change in the prevalence of pressure sores from the early 1990s compared to the late 1990s [48]. In the nursing home where there is an unparalleled onus of regulations, additional regulation is more likely to negatively affect patient care rather than accomplish the goal of improved pain management [49].

Nursing homes must maintain above 80% occupancy to have a positive balance sheet. Close economic margins have limited the ability to hire new staff as nursing homes struggle to remain solvent. Regulations are costly and time-consuming. Rarely is there a mechanism in place to evaluate the efficacy and burden of regulations once implemented. If ineffective, a mechanism should be in place to subsequently drop such regulations. Nursing homes continue to see costs escalate (in part due to a continual onslaught of new regulatory requirement and surveys) without funding to accommodate the additional financial burden. Genesis Health Ventures, Inc. initially filed for Chap. 11 in U.S. Court on June 22, 2002. Shortly after emerging from bankruptcy, the company's CEO resigned in mid-2002, indicating the need for work to reform nursing-home reimbursement, and reportedly remarked, "We need a permanent stable funding source for this industry to continue to exist. If Congress does nothing, the industry will collapse [50]." The significance of those words was amplified later that year as Genesis again experienced familiar financial difficulties and reportedly sought to sell off much of its nursing-home business.

In the pain field, the damage of overregulation has been impressive. The money wasted in association with State, Federal, and system regulatory requirements consists not only of taxes and revenue taken directly from the citizens and consumers to pay bureaucrats who oversee the regulations but also of indirect costs associated with lost energy that goes into filling out forms and the costs related to the distraction of creative power and diversion away from pain evaluation [51]. In most regulatory settings, the state surveyors have little to hold them accountable for decisions that are too frequently arbitrary, capricious, and fail to meet even cursory standards of proof. Also, there is little to ensure that regulators have adequate knowledge and experience in the nursing-home arena.

Conclusion

Pain does not exempt any population or any setting. Older adults are particularly susceptible to the grips of pain. If not by further regulation, how is pain relief to be fostered? The final chapter of this book, which deals with "Suggestions for change...," addresses this further. Recognition of the problem is the first step to resolution. For many physicians as well as other health-care professionals, the reason to enter medicine was primarily motivated by a desire to relieve suffering. Regrettably, data presented in this chapter and elsewhere indicate that all too often, the health-care professionals fail in resolving pain, one of the clearest factors associated with suffering. This is especially true when the person in pain is a senior. Sympathy and compassion are essential, but saying "I feel your pain" does not provide resolution. While recognizing and acknowledging that pain exists is necessary, it is not sufficient. There must also be proper assessment and, of course, proper intervention. Even this approach is incomplete. To be complete, there must also be attention to the prevention of pain. The chapters that follow in this edition of *The Handbook for Pain Relief in Older Adults* provide a comprehensive approach to help relieve suffering and to facilitate comfort.

References

1. Davis GC. Chronic pain management of older adults in residential settings. J Gerontol Nurs. 1997;23:16–22.
2. Crook J, Rideout E, Browne G. The prevalence of pain complaints among a general population. Pain. 1984;18:299–314.
3. Anderson S, Worm-Pederson J. The prevalence of persistent pain in a Danish population. In: Proc. 5th world congress on pain. Pain Suppl. 1987;4:s332.
4. Magni G, Marchetti M, Moreschi C, et al. Chronic musculoskeletal pain and depressive symptoms in the national health and nutrition examination. I. Epidemiologic follow-up study. Pain. 1993;53:163–8.
5. Cooner E, Amorosi S. The study of pain and older Americans. New York: Louis Harris and Associates; 1997.
6. Roy R, Michael T. A survey of chronic pain in an elderly population. Can Fam Physician. 1986;32:513–6.
7. Lau-Ting C, Phoon WO. Aches and pains among Singapore elderly. Singapore Med J. 1988;29:164–167.
8. Ferrell BA, Ferrell BR, Osterweil D. Pain in the nursing home. J Am Geriatr Soc. 1990;38:409–14.
9. Sengstaken EA, King SA. The problems of pain and its detection among geriatric nursing home residents. J Am Geratr Soc. 1993;41:541–4.
10. Won A, Lapane K, Gambassi G, et al. Correlates and management of nonmalignant pain in the nursing home. J Am Geriatr Soc. 1999;47:936–42.
11. Teno JM, Weitzen S, Wetle T, Mor V. Persistent pain in nursing home residents. JAMA. 2001;285:2081.
12. Cleeland CS, Gonin R, Hatfield AK, et al. Pain and its treatment in outpatients with metastatic cancer. N Engl J Med. 1994;330:592–6.

13. Landi F, Onder G, Cesari M, et al. Pain management in frail, community-living elderly patients. Arch Intern Med. 2001;161:2721–4.
14. AGS Panel on Chronic Pain in Older Persons. The management of chronic pain in older persons. American Geriatrics Society. J Am Geriatr Soc. 1998;46:635–51.
15. Reich J, Tupin J, Abromovitz S. Psychiatric diagnosis of chronic pain patients. Am J Psychiatry. 1983;140:1495–8.
16. Reid MC, Zhenchao G, Towle VR, et al. Pain-related disability among older male veterans receiving primary care. J Gerontol Med Sci. 2002;57A:M727–32.
17. . Turk D, Rudy T, Steig R. Pain and depression, I facts. Pain management; Nov–Dec 17–26, 1987.
18. Block AR, Kremer EF, Gaylor M. Behavioral treatment of chronic pain: the spouse as a discriminative cue for pain behavior. Pain. 1980;9:243–51.
19. Maroney C, Meier D, Moore C, Siu A, Litke A, Morrison RS. Gender differeces in reporting of pain and response to treatment in hospitalized patients. J Palliat Med. 2002; 5:207 (Abst #301).
20. Averbuch M, Katzper M. A search for sex differences in response to analgesia. Arch Intern Med. 2000;160:3424–8.
21. Gloth III FM. Geriatric pain: factors that limit pain relief and increase complications. Geriatrics. 2000;55(10):46–54.
22. Gloth III FM, Loury M. Complications of geriatric head and neck surgery. In: Eisele D, editor. Complications of head and neck surgery. Philadelphia, PA: B.C. Decker; 1993.
23. Crook J, Rodeout E, Browne G. The prevalence of pain complaints in a general population. Pain. 1984;18:299–314.
24. Nurmikko TJ. Postherpetic neuralgia: a model for neuropathic pain. In: Hansson P, Fields H, Hill R, Marchettini P, editors. Neuropathic pain: pathophysiology and treatment, progress in pain research and management. vol. 21. Seattle, WA: IASP; 2001. p. 151–67.
25. Abresch RT, Carter GT, Jensen MP, Kilmer DD. Assessment of pain and health-related quality of life in slowly progressive neuromuscular disease. Am J Hosp Palliat Care. 2002;19:39–48.
26. Lawrence RC, Helmick CG, Arnett FC, et al. Estimates of the prevalence of arthritis and selected musculoskeletal disorders in the United States. Arthritis Rheum. 1998;41:778–99.
27. Limcangco R. University of Maryland Doctoral Thesis; 2005.
28. Bond MR, Bonica JJ, Boyd DB, et al. For the International Association for the Study of Pain Subcommittee on Taxonomy. Classification of chronic pain: descriptions of chronic pain syndromes and definitions of pain terms. Pain. 1986;(Suppl 3):S216–21.
29. Rochon PA, Fortin PR, Dear KB, et al. Reporting of age data in clinical trials of arthritis. Deficiencies and solutions. Arch Intern Med. 1993;153:243–8.
30. Ferrell BA. Pain evaluation and management in the nursing home. Ann Intern Med. 1995;123:681–7.
31. Von Roenn JH, Cleeland CS, Gonin R, et al. Physician attitudes and practice in cancer pain management. A survey from the Eastern Cooperative Oncology Group. Ann Intern Med. 1993;119:121–6.
32. Hitchcock LS, Ferrell BR, McCaffery M. The experience of chronic non-malignant pain. J Pain Symptom Manage. 1994;9:312–8.
33. Gloth III FM. Pain management in older adults: prevention and treatment. J Am Geriatr Soc. 2001;49:188–99.
34. Sloan PA, et al. Cancer pain education among family physicians. J Pain Symptom Manage. 1997;14:74–81.
35. Breitbart W, Rosenfeld B, Passik SD. The network project: a multidisciplinary cancer education and training program in pain management, rehabilitation, and psychosocial issues. J Pain Symptom Manage. 1998;15:18–26.
36. Vortherms R, Ryan P, Ward S. Knowledge of, attitudes toward, and barriers to pharmacologic management of cancer pain in a statewide random sample of nurses. Res Nurs Health. 1992;15:459–66.

37. Portenoy RK, Payne R. Acute and chronic pain. In: Lowinson JH, Ruiz P, Millman RB, editors. Substance abuse: a comprehensive textbook. 2nd ed. Baltimore: Williams & Wilkins; 1992. p. 691–721.
38. Porter J, Jick H. Addiction rate in patients treated with narcotics. N Engl J Med. 1980;302:123.
39. Hendler N, Cimini C, Ma T, Tryba M. A comparison of cognitive impairment due to benzo-diazepines and to narcotics. Am J Psychiatry. 1980;137:828–30.
40. Vainio A, Ollila J, Matikainen E, Rosenberg P, Kaiso E. Driving ability in cancer patients receiving long-term morphine analgesia. Lancet. 1995;346:667–70.
41. AGS Panel on Persistent Pain in Older Persons. Pharmacological management of persistent pain in older persons. J Am Geriatr Soc. 2009;57(8):1331–46.
42. Weiner DK, Rudy TE. Attitudinal barriers to effective treatment of persistent pain in nursing home residents. J Am Geriatr Soc. 2002;50:2035–40.
43. Baran RW; For the Expert Panel. Guidelines for the management of chronic nonmalignant pain in the elderly LTC resident: the relief paradigm – part I. Long-term Care Interf. 2000;1(4):51–60.
44. American Medical Directors Association. Chronic pain management in the long-term care setting. Columbia, MD: American Medical Directors Association; 1999.
45. Ellison NM, McPherson ML, McGuire L. Pain report. Dannemiller Memorial Educational Foundation pain report: an update on issues, research and treatment trends. Enhanced Marketing, Ltd. 2000;1(1):1–3.
46. Zerzan J, Stearns S, Hanson L. Access to palliative care and hospice in nursing homes. JAMA. 2000;284:2489–94.
47. Pitkala KH, Strandberg TE, Reijo ST. Management of nonmalignant pain in home-dwelling older people: a population-based survey. J Am Geriatr Soc. 2002;50:1861–5.
48. Coleman EA, Martau JM, Lin MK, Kramer AM. Pressure ulcer prevalence in long-term nursing home residents since the implementation of OBRA'87. J Am Geriatr Soc. 2002;50:728–32.
49. Thompson TG. Report to congress: appropriateness of minimum nurse staffing ratios in nursing homes phase II final report. From the Center for Medicare and Medicaid Services Website. http://www.cms.gov/medicaid/reports/rp1201home.asp Updated June 12, 2002.
50. Goldstein J. Genesis health ventures CEO resigns. Posted on the world wide web by the Philadelphia inquirer on May 29, 2002 at http://www.philly.com/mld/inquirer/living/health/3356552.htm.
51. Stossel J. The real cost of regulation. Imprimis. 2001;30(5):1–5.

Chapter 3
Assessment

F. Michael Gloth, III

You can't fix it, if you can't measure it.

Demming

It was a sunny afternoon in an ocean resort town in Maryland. A physician was seeing routine patients when a young man in his 30s walked into the office complaining of back pain. The patient was new to the office and after a 20-min visit left with a prescription for 20 tablets of oxycodone. What did not come out in the brief cursory history that the physician had obtained was that the man was an undercover agent and part of a sting operation. A few months later the case came before the Maryland Board of Physicians. The physician had written the prescription for this new patient without ever performing an examination or a formal assessment of pain. Few people would argue about the inappropriateness of the physician's actions, and it took little time for the largest adjudicatory board in the nation to relieve that physician of his license. Even when a clinician elicits some history and a physical examination, too often an analgesic is prescribed without a formal assessment of pain status. This clinically common practice of inadequate pain assessment is responsible for much of the inadequacy of pain management [1]. One can speculate on many reasons to explain the deficits in practice. Every clinician learns how to do a blood pressure, oftentimes before entering the school of their profession. For pain, there is not a standard scale that serves each population well. Only recently have medical schools started to incorporate formal instruction in pain assessment.

Of course, evaluation of pain must go beyond the measurement obtained with a good pain assessment instrument. Assessing pain in seniors also involves a careful history and physical examination as well as clinical testing as indicated based on the results of the initial clinical findings. To successfully manage pain, all elements of the assessment must be present and done well. This chapter explores the concept of

F.M. Gloth, III(✉)
Division of Geriatric Medicine and Gerontology, Johns Hopkins University
School of Medicine, Baltimore, MD, USA
e-mail: fgloth1@jhmi.edu

F.M. Gloth, III (ed.), *Handbook of Pain Relief in Older Adults: An Evidence-Based Approach*, Aging Medicine, DOI 10.1007/978-1-60761-618-4_3,
© Springer Science+Business Media, LLC 2011

assessment instruments that often provide the first line of screening for the presence of pain. A discussion of the other important elements of history and physical examination is warranted here. Throughout, it should be emphasized that the assessment process must also weigh the efficacy and safety of every intervention as importantly as discovering the presence of pain in the first place. In other words, evaluation must incorporate potential options that will be acceptable to the individual in pain. If a test is designed to determine whether a surgical intervention is necessary, but the patient is not a surgical candidate, then the test itself is likely to be unwarranted.

A site principal investigator at a research conference was overheard saying, "A pain scale is a pain scale…They're all no good." As the comment suggests, adequate standardization for pain scales is oftentimes lacking. For blood pressure instruments, standardization is commonplace and instruments come to market with relative accuracy and precision. Standardization of pain scales is far more complex due to the subjective nature of such instruments. Because of subpopulation variability, it only makes sense that pain scales used in older adults should be tested in older adults. Ideally, there should be some evidence that an instrument is valid and reliable and importantly, responsive (sensitive to changes) for pain. The user also must recognize that some flexibility must exist for pain scales. Institutions that insist on a single pain scale in all settings, in the interest of uniformity, do a disservice to the clinician and to the people suffering with pain. For older individuals who have visual impairment, the visual analogue scales or those with facial expressions to reflect various pain levels are impractical. Despite the likelihood of having visually impaired patients, many health care institutions will still favor one scale throughout the facility, which incorporates such vision-dependent concepts [2]. Ideally, a scale will be standardized in a population with similar characteristics as the individual patient being assessed.

Selecting Pain Scales for Seniors

Few scales have been developed specifically with older individuals in mind. Surprisingly, few have been evaluated for responsiveness, i.e., sensitivity to changes, in pain. Given the importance that hospitals and nursing homes are now mandated to place on pain assessment (and subsequent treatment and evaluation of that treatment), it is disconcerting that so many instruments to assess pain have not had such testing. Many scales are variations of an identical concept, i.e., one end with "no pain" and the other end with "very bad" pain (or some variation thereof). These scales use numbers, faces, thermometers, or simply lines [3, 4]. These scales are consistent in another way in that the speed with which they can be administered in an appropriate environment is relatively brief. It is vital to have instruments in a clinical environment that are standardized adequately and can be administered in less than a minute.

The Functional Pain Scale (FPS) [5] is one scale that can be administered easily and rapidly, has been designed for seniors, and has had appropriate standardization, including responsiveness testing. The FPS offers another advantage. It has an objective component that handles confounding, when patients selecting the highest level on a pain scale regardless of changes (improvements) that occur in pain status. This sometimes happens when patients fear that analgesia will be scaled back should they achieve any degree of relief. It is easy to rationalize why such a phenomenon may occur. Inadequate pain control and analgesia administration go hand-in-hand. A patient who has experienced inconsistency in getting adequate analgesia may be reluctant to acknowledge improvement in pain due to anxiety about not maintaining sufficient medication. A physician colleague who had been in a severe motor vehicle accident with extensive trauma confided his reluctance in ever reporting his pain level at less than a "7" on a 10-point scale due to fear that his analgesics, which had finally started to provide some pain relief, would be decreased or even stopped. This was from someone who had extraordinary access to some of the most recognized physicians in the world! It is easy to understand how other patients might be moved to inflate their pain scale scores as well.

Regardless of the reasoning process, such manipulation provides a dilemma for the well-versed clinician who recognizes the importance of listening to patients, especially when describing pain. However, when a patient who, an hour earlier was writhing in bed unable participate in providing a history due to excruciating pain, now appears calm and reports that the pain is "still a ten" in between bites of dinner, the utility of a 0–10 scale may come under question in that specific circumstance. The FPS provides some objective components, which augment a traditional, purely subjective, numerical scale. For example, the highest level of pain on the FPS (see Fig. 3.1) is categorized as pain so intense that one is unable to communicate because of the pain. This, of course, precludes anyone from consistently stating that the pain is at the highest level. The objective nature of the other functional components may contribute to understanding why this scale outperforms other scales in responsiveness, including the McGill Pain Questionnaire (Short form) and the Visual Analog Scale [5–7]. Another advantage of the FPS is that it has been tested in subjects with Mini-Mental State Examination© scores as low as 17, i.e., in those with severe dementia.

Some circumstances continue to perplex clinicians trying to evaluate pain levels. Assessing the heavily subjective level of pain in an individual who has markedly impaired communicative capacity or who is otherwise cognitively impaired can be enigmatic. The bulk of publications related to this issue are found in the nursing literature [8, 9]. Unfortunately, attempts to meet this challenge have not produced a definitive solution. Ideally, such scales would be studied in a population that is cognitively intact and unable to communicate for a transient period of time. A transient ischemic attack that does not affect memory would be such a circumstance. Such a study would be extremely difficult, because of the inability to predict when someone is going to have such an event or timing the assessment during the transient event. Operations that render an individual unable to verbally communicate, or assessing individuals involved in dental procedures, may be somewhat helpful in the design of worthwhile trials. One also would like to standardize such instruments in a population that is cognitively impaired and unable to verbally communicate. Validation and responsiveness testing is particularly daunting in such circumstances.

FUNCTIONAL PAIN SCALE

0 = No Pain

1 = Tolerable (and does not prevent any activities)

2 = Tolerable (but does prevent some activities)

3 = Intolerable (but can use telephone, watch TV, or read)

4 = Intolerable (but can't use a telephone, watch TV, or read because of pain)

5 = Intolerable (and unable to verbally communicate because of pain)

Ideally all patients should reach a 0-2 level, preferably 0-1. It should be made clear to the respondent that limitations in function only apply if limitations are due to the pain being evaluated.

May be reproduced for clinical purposes. NB: Where a 0-10 scale is desired consider modification as follows: replace 0, 1, 2, 3, 4, 5, with 0, 1, 3, 5, 7, 10 respectively.

Fig. 3.1 The Functional Pain Scale achieves a score from 0 to 5 based on subjective and objective question responses related to whether pain is tolerable and whether it interferes with some activities

Assessment of Pain When Communication Is Impaired

When pain is suspected in a person who is unable to verbally communicate, or understand, such as the case with receptive aphasia often seen after strokes, the assessment of pain will depend heavily on being able to recognize aberrant physical or behavioral responses [10, 11]. Body language that has typically been associated with pain, unfortunately also may be associated with other etiologies. For example, grimacing or wincing may be associated with nausea, disgust, or distaste. Fist clenching or muscle tightening may be associated with anger. Withdrawal can be reflexic and/or occur with being frightened or startled, or even in response to tickling. Crying can, of course, reflect sadness, or in many circumstances, even happiness.

Usually, adequate assessment in a person who is unable to communicate includes a best guess assessment of common body language and behavioral manifestations, in conjunction with a trial intervention, which may or may not include drugs. Distinguishing the usual from unusual responses may play an important role in such pain assessment. Reassessment to determine whether the behavior or physical

Table 3.1 Table of pain assessment tools for nonverbal patients (Direct Observation Instruments)

The Pain Assessment in Advanced Dementia (PAINAD) Scale, (Warden et al., 2003)

Checklist of Nonverbal Pain Indicators (CNPI), (Feldt, 2000)

The Pain Assessment Scale for Seniors with Severe Dementia-Dutch (PACSLAC-D)
  (Zwakhalen, Hamers & Bergen, 2007)

Mobilization–Observation–Behavior–Intensity–Dementia Pain Scale (MOBID)
  (Husebo et al., 2007)

Nursing Assistant-Administered Instrument to Assess Pain in Demented Individuals (NOPPAIN)
  (Snow et al., 2004)

Pain Behaviors for Osteoarthritis Instrument for Cognitively Impaired Elders (PBOICIE)
  (Tsai et al., 2008)

manifestation has been modified is also important. In the noncommunicating patient, a high index of clinical suspicion, combined with close observation for changes associated with any interventions, will be the key to successful pain control. Some scales for nonverbal patients are listed in Table 3.1.

Research vs. Clinical Care Instruments

It is useful to consider that, like many things in life, the most commonly used items are not necessarily the best ones. Pain assessment tools that are commonly used are likely to be more commonly used because people have been exposed to them. Thus, assessment instruments that get a lot of exposure in the literature are more likely to be used. Instruments that are most likely to get such exposure are instruments that are developed by people who are experts and publish or speak a great deal. On the other hand, many would argue that people who write a great deal are, by the virtue of writing on a topic, thus perceived as experts. Some of this is explored in more detail in the chapter on the Politics of Pain. In essence, it is important to evaluate the standardization and the applicability of each pain scale instrument as it relates to the population undergoing assessment.

To illustrate this concept further consider the following set of events, which actually occurred. A conversation with a colleague revealed that her division had recently switched pain assessment tools because validity data seemed to be better in studies of populations similar to their clinic population. To the dismay of this colleague, the division had switched back to the old scale because it was so commonly used in studies in the rheumatology field. There was concern that studies submitted for review might be jeopardized by using a scale that was less common or less familiar to potential reviewers. At a bureaucratic level, the fundamental importance was on recognition of an instrument rather than on the quality of the pain assessment.

Just as important as validation or reliability is the concept of responsiveness or sensitivity to changes in levels of pain. Since the Joint Commission for Accreditation of Hospital Organizations (JCAHO) and other organizations have begun to monitor for the assessment of pain and whether the interventions instituted have had an impact on pain level, assessment tools that can identify changes in levels of pain are becoming more desirable. Scales that have not demonstrated utility in populations being assessed should generate some concern, as should those that have not had responsiveness testing, even if they have been around for a long period of time.

As noted above, administering an analgesic without formally assessing pain is relatively common, and inadequate assessment is strongly associated with inadequate pain management [12]. For many reasons, assessment tools may not be routinely used. Since few have been adequately tested in older adults, it is difficult to determine the appropriate instrument in that population. Pain scales standardized in a younger population may not be as helpful in seniors. For example, a scale that uses changes from a "smiley face" to one with a frown was developed for children and may not be acceptable to the recently retired company president. Conversely, the older individual is more likely to have achieved a lower education level, which makes some assessment tools that use words like "lancinating" less helpful in assessing pain levels and, importantly, in measuring any change in pain [13].

Delirium and dementia can also be barriers to pain assessment [14]. An experience with an older adult who had early dementia with loss of some executive function demonstrated the shortcomings of the Visual Analog Scale as he responded that his pain was "…not on the line," but in his shoulder.

Pain assessment and management, particularly, in a frail, elderly population remain difficult due to the subjective nature of pain and the limitations of ascertaining pain levels in a consistent manner. The psychometric properties of pain scales frequently have not been tested in seniors. This is combined with the fact that more prevalent visual and cognitive deficits may make it difficult to use some instruments in this population [15]. Many patients fail to comprehend such questions, which ask them to rate their pain on a linear scale, but can more easily determine if their pain interferes with their functional ability. By testing patients' level of pain with respect to its interference with their daily function, a more accurate measure of their pain may be ascertained.

The nature of the older population makes testing such instruments challenging. For example, any reliability testing (In other words, "Will the assessment instrument perform well, consistently, and regardless of who is administering it?") is dependent on reproducible performance in a stable study cohort. It should be recognized, however, that finding a frail older population that has a stable pain status is quite challenging [16].

It should also be noted that a scale may perform well in healthy subjects, but when administered to a smaller subset that may be more typical of the population likely to need such scales, less impressive results are attained. For example, it was noted that two patients claimed to be unable to rate their pain on the Present Pain Intensity scale, during a comparison trial in evaluating the FPS, yet were able to give a score on the FPS. Such anecdotal events might suggest real differences in a typical subset of the frail elderly population that frequently will present with pain complaints. Vigilance of clinicians and researchers toward detecting deficiencies in scales that rate well with large populations, but fall short with subpopulations of interest is warranted.

Another potential problem with some pain scales currently in practice is the length of time needed to administer them. Ideally, any pain assessment tool for clinical use will involve a measurement that can be taken quickly (usually less than a minute), something that is important for an individual in a great deal of pain who may not have the patience to choose from a list of 80 words to describe their anguish. Celerity in administration is also a property that the busy clinician will find appealing in today's hectic pace of medical practice.

Some tools are easily misused by clinical staff, who are not adequately educated on administration of tools preferred in one institution versus another. For example, a nurse who worked in multiple clinical settings and was unfamiliar with the Faces Pain Scale held the scale up by the patient and rated the pain based on the image that most closely resembled the expression on the patient's face. Regrettably, this is a surprisingly common phenomenon in patients who are unable to verbally communicate. For this reason, the Faces Pain Scale may be better avoided in settings where frequent supervision and administration instruction can be provided to staff.

Beyond Screening Instruments

Beyond that initial (and subsequent) evaluation with a good pain assessment tool, the management direction will be predicated upon a good clinical history of the pain and a competent physical examination. In seniors, both are likely to take more time than in younger patients, if only because seniors are unlikely to follow Ocham's razor (multiple complaints are likely caused by a single diagnosis), i.e., for seniors, multiple problems may contribute to even a single complaint.

The history must involve basic elements that include location, timing, ameliorating and exacerbating factors, context, duration, quality, severity, and any associated signs or symptoms. It should also be noted that some people would deny "pain" but admit to "discomfort," an "ache," or some similar terminology for pain [17].

Location should involve not only the area of the body, but whether the pain is superficial or deep. The pain may also be localized to bone, joint, muscle, etc. Location here does not refer to pain that may accompany change in physical or geographic location, e.g., accompanying rapid transitions to high altitudes, rapid changes in depths when diving, or visits to certain relatives or ceremonial dinners, all of which might be more properly categorized as "modifying factors." (In the case of certain relatives and ceremonial dinners, some might argue that they would be better categorized as the *cause* of pain…)

Timing includes whether the pain is continuous or intermittent. If intermittent, when does it occur, for example, upon awakening? If continuous, are there times when it is worse than others? Regardless of whether continuous or intermittent, modifying factors need to be determined. Recognizing that pain frequently occurs immediately after physical therapy sessions may be an indication for preemptive analgesia, modification of the therapy regimen, or both.

Whether the pain occurs in certain settings and the overall context of the pain, e.g., postoperatively or as part of a chronic or persistent scenario, are also important pieces of information. Determining whether it interferes with specific activities or functions also should be documented. Does the pain limit social activity, appetite, sleep, intimacy, or other factors impacting quality of life?

The duration refers to the acute or chronic nature of the pain. Pain that has been present for months or years may have different etiologies as well as different associated symptoms. Additionally, the approach to chronic or persistent pain may be different than acute or transient pain situations.

Associated signs and symptoms may refer directly to the pain etiology but also to comorbid findings, e.g., depressive symptoms. Changes in function also may accompany pain. Thus, an assessment of function using an appropriately standardized instrument for the senior being evaluated is warranted [18, 19].

The quality of the pain, i.e., burning, dull, throbbing, shock-like, tearing, and other such descriptors must be ascertained as well. Severity must accompany the rest of the history. Usually, here is where a score on a specified pain scale will be documented. Other subjective terms may appear here as well.

It is also important to recognize and document observations about secondary gain, anxiety, prior experiences, mental focus, and other psychological factors that may impact pain status. Spiritual issues and social support should also be recognized as important factors that should be identified in the history [20]. A later chapter in this book (by Dr. Mulligan et al.) deals specifically with spirituality, which is infrequently described and often has a tremendous impact on pain management.

A good social history will include information on an older patient's social support structure. This will provide valuable information with regards to ability to attend therapy sessions that may require transportation, accessibility to pharmacies, and financial capabilities that bear on prescription coverage and other such factors associated with medication and treatment options. It makes little sense to develop a treatment plan without knowing whether the patient can feasibly comply. Provided that the patient is agreeable, it also may be useful to involve other family members who may be sources of such support and who can help provide such information.

A good medication history, especially what has been tried and proven problematic or ineffective, can be very helpful when ultimately developing a treatment plan. So too, will be information on patient concerns. For example, a patient who fears addiction or does not believe that notification of pain will produce relief may be reluctant to comply with recommendations [21].

Advance directives, including the designation of the health care agent to render decisions should the patient not be able to do so, are a necessary part of the history. This should ideally be obtained early during a routine visit setting. Remember that this is a decision that, for many patients, will require the input of other people with whom the patient places confidence. Thus, while the discussion should be initiated, it may be only temporarily resolved until a later visit after more input can be obtained.

Recognizing that many older patients see several physicians because of multiple comorbid conditions, it is important to identify that any other clinicians involved in the patient's care. It is also useful to determine which clinicians are responsible for which therapies. Such information will facilitate communication among clinicians during efforts to modify regimens and when working on the task of medicinal debridement, i.e., reducing the number and frequency of medications, for patients with polypharmacy issues.

The physical examination in the older population requires additional diligence as well. Seniors may present with different symptoms than their younger counterparts. For example, visceral pain may be less intense in the seniors and, even serious infectious causes of pain may have minimal or absent leukocytosis [22]. Even presentations of pain, e.g., headache, which is common and usually benign in young patients, may be due to more serious causes for older patients. For example, the headache in an older adult is more likely to be associated with etiologies such as temporal arteritis, cervical osteoarthritis, depression, congestive heart failure, subdural hematoma, or electrolyte disturbances [23].

The physical examination should, of course, include the site of reported pain, common areas for pain referral, and common sites of pain in older patients [24]. In addition to an evaluation for tenderness, other aspects of the examination should look for clues pointing to the major underlying diagnostic basis. Thus, erythema, neurologic abnormalities, functional decline are all clinical findings that may help in ascertaining a root cause of pain and the impact on quality of life. It should be mentioned that whether function is measured by a performance-based tool or not, the instrument selected should have the same type of standardization and responsiveness testing described for pain scales above [19]. Additionally, the examination should also encompass physical changes that might be induced by the pain itself. For example, favoring a painful knee may induce malalignment of the spine, exacerbation of osteoarthritis in the opposite knee, and similar changes due to adjustments made consciously or unconsciously in response to the painful joint. The abnormal elements of the physical examination should be clearly documented at baseline and followed serially as treatment progresses.

For the patient who has been treated with opioids for pain, the physical examination should also be performed with the astute clinician mindful of the potential for drug withdrawal. In older adults, addiction is rarely an issue. A far greater problem is having patients decrease medications or even completely discontinue medications for pain without discussing such changes with the physician. As pain improves, patients will decide that the opioid, which they had been fearful of starting in the first place because of concerns about addiction or because of reading an unrelated story about abuse potential, is no longer needed. Subsequently, agitation, tremulousness, and, often, more pain develop among other signs and symptoms associated with opioid withdrawal.

In addition to those elements of the physical examination directed toward discovering the direct etiology of pain and the changes associated with such pain, the examination in seniors must include elements that will affect communication and compliance with intervention strategies as well. Therefore, an examination of hearing and vision is crucial. For seniors, aging is associated with loss in high frequency tones as well as difficulty in sound discrimination. This combined with other causes of hearing loss may make comprehension of instructions for pain control difficult. Presbyopia, age-related difficulty in focusing on close objects, and other causes of visual impairment may make reading prescriptions and small print impossible. Distinguishing among the expressions on the Faces Pain Scale also may not be reasonable.

An assessment of cognitive function is also needed. Such assessments should include an evaluation of executive function. Appropriate tests for baseline evaluation will be important and including acceptable measures to monitor changes in such functioning will also be required. It should be noted that other sensory deficits may increase the risk for mental status changes as well [25–27]. As part of the cognitive assessment, screening and evaluation for depression is particularly important since depression is not only common, but pain is very difficult to adequately treat, if depression is not also adequately treated [28].

In summary, the assessment of pain in older adults is absolutely vital, if one is to be successful in resolving pain. The assessment should involve formal assessment instruments, preferably standardized in populations similar to the individual who is being assessed. A good history and physical examination by an astute clinician must also be part of pain assessment. While the frustration of the physician quoted at the beginning of this chapter is understandable, it should be recognized that pain scales do differ. Nonetheless, there remains great room for research to improve the understanding of appropriate use of those currently in existence and to develop new scales for populations not adequately served by currently available assessment modalities.

References

1. Von Roenn JH, Cleeland CS, Gonin R, Hatfield AK, Pandya KJ. Physician attitudes and practice in cancer pain management. A survey from the Eastern Cooperative Oncology Group. Ann Intern Med. 1993;119:121–6.
2. Weiner DK, Hanlon JT. Pain in nursing home residents. Drugs Aging. 2001;18:13–29.
3. Joint Commission on Accreditation of Healthcare Organizations. Pain assessment and management: an organizational approach. Oakbrook Terrace, IL: Joint Commission; 2000. p. 15.
4. The AGS Panel on Persistent Pain in Older Persons. The management of persistent pain in older adults. J Am Geriatr Soc. 2002;50 Suppl 6:S209.
5. Gloth FM 3rd, Scheve AA, Stober CV, Chow S, Prosser J.. The *Functional Pain Scale* (FPS): reliability, validity, and responsiveness in a senior population. J Am Med Dir Assoc. 2001;2(3):110–4.
6. Herr KA, Mobily PR, Kohout FJ, Wagenaar D. Evaluation of the Faces Pain Scale for use with the elderly. Clin J Pain. 1998;14:29–38.
7. Briggs M, Closs JS. A descriptive study of the use of visual analogue scales and verbal rating scales for the assessment of postoperative pain in orthopedic patients. J Pain Symptom Manage. 1999;18:438–46.
8. Miller J, Neelon V, Dalton J, et al. The assessment of discomfort in elderly confused patients: a preliminary study. J Neurosci Nurs. 1996;28:175–82.

9. Wynne CF, Ling SM, Remsburg R. Comparison of pain assessment instruments in cognitively intact and cognitively impaired nursing home residents. Geriatr Nurs. 2000;21:20–3.
10. Gaston-Johansson F, Johansson F, Johansson C. Pain in the elderly, prevalence, attitudes, and nursing assessment. Ann LTC. 1996;4:325–31.
11. American Medical Directors Association Consensus Panel. Clinical practice guidelines for chronic pain management in the long-term care setting. Columbia, MD: American Medical Directors Association; 1999.
12. Von Roenn JH, Cleeland CS, Gonin R, Hatfield AK, Pandya KJ. Physician attitudes and practice in cancer pain management. A survey from the Eastern Cooperative Oncology Group. Ann Intern Med. 1993;119:121–6.
13. Melzack R.. The McGill Pain Questionnaire: major properties and scoring methods. Pain. 1975;1:277–99.
14. Kane RL, Ouslander JG, Abrass IB, editors. Essentials of clinical geriatrics. 2nd ed. New York: McGraw Hill; 1989.
15. U.S. Department of Health & Human Services. AHCPR Clinical Practice Guidelines; Management of Cancer Pain. No. 94-0592; March 1994. p. 129.
16. Weiner et al. Predictors of pain self-report in nursing home residents. Aging Clin Exp Res 1998; 10:411–20.
17. Miller J, Neelon V, Dalton J, Ng'andu N, Bailey D Jr, Layman E, et al. The assessment of discomfort in elderly confused patients: a preliminary study. J Neurosci Nurs. 1996;28:175–82.
18. Gloth FM 3rd, Walston JD, Meyers JM, Pearson J. Reliability and validity of the Frail Elderly Functional Assessment (FEFA) questionnaire. Am J Phys Med Rehabil. 1995;74(1):45–53.
19. Gloth FM 3rd, Scheve AA, Shah S, Ashton R, McKinney R. Responsiveness and validity in alternative settings for the Frail Elderly Functional Assessment (FEFA) questionnaire. Arch Phys Med Rehab. 1999;80:1572–6.
20. Krause et al. Church-based support and health in old age. J Gerontol. 2002;57A:S332–47.
21. Weiner D, et al. Attitudinal barriers to effective treatment of persistent pain in the nursing home. J Am Geriatr Soc. 2002;50:2035–40.
22. Marco CA, Schoenfeld CN, Keyl PM, Menkes ED, Doehring MC. Abdominal pain in geriatric emergency patients: variables associated with adverse outcomes. Acad Emerg Med. 1998;5:1163–8.
23. Gordon RS. Pain in the elderly. JAMA. 1979;241:2491–2.
24. The AGS Panel on Persistent Pain in Older Persons. The management of persistent pain in older adults. J Am Geriatr Soc. 2002;50 Suppl 6:S205–24.
25. Uhlmann RF, Teri L, Rees TS, et al. Impact of hearing loss on mental status testing. J Am Geriatr Soc. 1989;37:223–8.
26. Uhlmann RF, Larson EB, Rees TS, et al. Relationship of hearing impairment to dementia. JAMA. 1989;261:1916–9.
27. Gennis V, Garry PJ, Haaland KY, et al. Hearing and cognition in the elderly. Arch Int Med. 1991;151:2259–64.
28. Parmelee PA, Katz IR, Lawton MP. The relation of pain to depression among institutionalized aged. J Gerontol. 1991;46:P15–21.

Chapter 4
AGS 2009 Guidelines for Pharmacological Management of Persistent Pain in Older Adults

F. Michael Gloth, III

Pharmacologic agents remain the most commonly utilized strategy for pain management in older individuals... Furthermore, a comprehensive approach to treatment that combines both pharmacologic and nonpharmacologic approaches is recommended.

2009 AGS Guidelines on Pharmacological Management of Persistent Pain in Older Persons

Pharmacological Guidance for Pain Management in Older Adults

In 1998, the American Geriatrics Society (AGS) published their first guideline on managing pain in older adults. Since then, two additional guidelines have been published to update clinicians on the management of persistent pain in older adults. The most recent of these was recently released in 2009, as Guidelines for Pharmacological Management of Persistent Pain in Older Adults [1, 2]. The most recent guidelines used a system of evaluation, called the Grading of Recommendations Assessment, Development, and Evaluation (GRADE). This system evaluates evidence in the literature based on degrees of quality and strength. Recommendations were subsequently made in accordance with the risks or benefits of using a pharmacotherapy couched with the weight of evidence in one direction or the other. Hence, weak recommendations were given in unclear circumstances where the benefits were balanced by approximately equal risks or where data where inadequate to place sufficient confidence in a strong recommendation. The recommendations appear below.

F.M. Gloth, III (✉)
Division of Geriatric Medicine and Gerontology, Johns Hopkins University
School of Medicine, Baltimore, MD, USA
e-mail: fgloth1@jhmi.edu

F.M. Gloth, III (ed.), *Handbook of Pain Relief in Older Adults: An Evidence-Based Approach*, Aging Medicine, DOI 10.1007/978-1-60761-618-4_4,
© Springer Science+Business Media, LLC 2011

Table 4.1 Key to Designations of Quality and Strength of Evidence[2]

Quality of Evidence	
High	Evidence includes consistent results from well-designed, well-conducted studies in representative populations that directly assess effects on health outcomes (at least two consistent, higher-quality randomized controlled trials or multiple, consistent observational studies with no significant methodological flaws showing large effects).
Moderate	Evidence is sufficient to determine effects on health outcomes, but the strength of the evidence is limited by the number, quality, size, or consistency of included studies, generalizability to routine practice, or indirect nature of the evidence on health outcomes (at least one higher quality trial with >100 subjects; two or more higher-quality trials with some inconsistency; at least two consistent, lower-quality trials, or multiple, consistent observational studies with no significant methodological flaws showing at least moderate effects).
Low	Evidence is insufficient to assess effects on health outcomes because of limited number or power of studies, large and unexplained inconsistency between higher quality studies, important flaws in study design or conduct, gaps in the chain of evidence, or lack of information on important health outcomes.
Strength of Recommendation	
Strong	Benefits clearly outweigh risks and burden OR risks and burden clearly outweigh benefits
Weak	Benefits finely balanced with risks and burden
Insufficient: "I" recommendation	Insufficient evidence to determine net benefits or risks

Specific Recommendations

(Quality and strength of evidence ratings follow each recommendation: see Table 4.1)

NSAIDs

I. Acetaminophen should be considered as initial and ongoing pharmacotherapy in the treatment of persistent pain, particularly musculoskeletal pain, owing to its demonstrated effectiveness and good safety profile (high quality of evidence; strong recommendation).

   A Absolute contraindications: liver failure (high quality of evidence, strong recommendation)

   B Relative contraindications and cautions: hepatic insufficiency, chronic alcohol abuse/dependence (moderate quality of evidence, strong recommendation)

   C Maximum daily recommended dosages should not be exceeded and must include "hidden sources" such as from combination pills (moderate quality of evidence, strong recommendation).

II. Nonselective NSAIDs and COX-2 selective inhibitors may be considered rarely, and with extreme caution, in highly selected individuals (high quality of evidence, strong recommendation).

   A Patient selection: other (safer) therapies have failed; evidence of continuing therapeutic goals met; ongoing assessment of risks/complications outweighed by therapeutic benefits (low quality of evidence, strong recommendation).

   B Absolute contraindications: current active peptic ulcer disease (low quality of evidence, strong recommendation), chronic kidney disease (moderate level of evidence, strong recommendation), and heart failure (moderate level of evidence, weak recommendation).

   C Relative contraindications and cautions: hypertension, *H. pylori*, history of peptic ulcer disease, concomitant use of steroids, or SSRIs (moderate quality of evidence, strong recommendation).

III. Older persons taking nonselective NSAIDs should use a proton pump inhibitor or misoprostol for gastrointestinal protection (high quality of evidence, strong recommendation).

IV. Patients taking a COX-2 selective inhibitor with aspirin should use a proton pump inhibitor or misoprostol for gastrointestinal protection (high quality of evidence, strong recommendation).

V. Patients should not take more than one nonselective NSAID/COX-2 selective inhibitor for pain control (low quality of evidence, strong recommendation).

VI. Patients taking ASA for cardioprophylaxis should not use ibuprofen (moderate quality of evidence, weak recommendation).

VII. All patients taking nonselective NSAIDs and COX-2 selective inhibitors should be routinely assessed for gastrointestinal and renal toxicity, hypertension, heart failure, and other drug–drug and drug–disease interactions (weak quality of evidence, strong recommendation).

Opioids

VIII. All patients with moderate–severe pain, pain-related functional impairment or diminished quality of life due to pain should be considered for opioid therapy (low quality of evidence, strong recommendation).

IX. Patients with frequent or continuous pain on a daily basis should be treated with ATC time-contingent dosing aimed at achieving steady-state opioid therapy (low quality of evidence, weak recommendation).

X. Clinicians should anticipate, assess for, and identify potential opioid-associated adverse effects (moderate quality of evidence, strong recommendation).

XI. Maximal safe doses of acetaminophen or NSAIDs should not be exceeded when using fixed-dose opioid combination agents as part of an analgesic regimen (moderate quality of evidence, strong recommendation).

XII. When long-acting opioid preparations are prescribed, breakthrough pain should be anticipated, assessed, prevented, and/or treated using short-acting immediate opioid medications (moderate quality of evidence, strong recommendation).

XIII. Methadone should be initiated and titrated cautiously only by clinicians well versed in its use and risks (moderate quality of evidence, strong recommendation).

XIV. Patients taking opioid analgesics should be reassessed for ongoing attainment of therapeutic goals, adverse effects, and safe and responsible medication use (moderate quality of evidence, strong recommendation).

Adjuvant

XV. All patients with neuropathic pain are candidates for adjuvant analgesics (strong quality of evidence, strong recommendation).

XVI. Patients with fibromyalgia are candidates for a trial of approved adjuvant analgesics (moderate quality of evidence, strong recommendation).

XVII. Patients with other types of refractory persistent pain may be candidates for certain adjuvant analgesics (e.g., back pain, headache, diffuse bone pain, and temporomandibular disorder) (low quality of evidence, weak recommendation).

XVIII. Tertiary tricyclic antidepressants (amitriptyline, imipramine, and doxepin) should be avoided because of higher risk for adverse effects (e.g., anticholinergic effects and cognitive impairment) (moderate quality of evidence, strong recommendation).

XIX. Agents may be used alone, but often the effects are enhanced when used in combination with other pain analgesics and/or nondrug strategies (moderate quality of evidence, strong recommendation).

XX. Therapy should begin with the lowest possible dose and increase slowly based on response and side effects, with the caveat that some agents have a delayed onset of action and therapeutic benefits are slow to develop. For example, gabapentin may require 2–3 weeks for onset of efficacy (moderate quality of evidence, strong recommendation).

XXI. An adequate therapeutic trial should be conducted before discontinuation of a seemingly ineffective treatment (weak quality of evidence, strong recommendation).

Other Drugs

XXII. Long-term systemic corticosteroids should be reserved only for patients with pain-associated inflammatory disorders or metastatic bone pain. Osteoarthritis should not be considered an inflammatory disorder (moderate quality of evidence, strong recommendation).

XXIII. All patients with localized neuropathic pain are candidates for topical lido-caine (moderate quality of evidence, strong recommendation).

XXIV. Patients with localized nonneuropathic pain may be candidates for topical lidocaine (low quality of evidence, weak recommendation).

XXV. All patients with other localized nonneuropathic persistent pain may be candidates for topical NSAIDs (moderate quality of evidence, weak recommendation).

XXVI. Other topical agents may be considered for regional pain syndromes including capsaicin or menthol (moderate quality of evidence, weak recommendation).

XXVII. Many other agents for specific pain syndromes may require caution in older persons and merit further research (e.g., glucosamine, chondroitin, cannabinoids, botulinum toxin, alpha-2 adrenergic agonists, calcitonin, vitamin D, bisphosphonates, and ketamine) (low quality of evidence, weak recommendation).

Like other recommendations, acetaminophen is recommended early in the phar-macologic algorithm. Nonsteroidal anti-inflammatory agents (NSAIDs) fit in the category of drugs to be avoided on a chronic basis. These guidelines were written prior to approval of agents with a nitrous oxide moiety. There is reason to believe that such drugs may offer a safer alternative to traditional NSAIDs. At the time of this writing, the Food and Drug Administration was considering, the first of such agents, niproxcinod, for approval. Topical agents were considered to be safer options for localized pain where oral NSAIDs might otherwise be considered.

A trial of opioid therapy for older patients with moderate-to-severe persistent pain was also recommended with guidance from two sets of questions.

I.

1. What is conventional practice for this type of pain or pain patient?
2. Is there an alternative therapy that is likely to have an equivalent or better therapeutic index for pain control, functional restoration, and improvement in quality of life?
3. Does the patient have medical problems that may increase the risk of opioid-related adverse effects?
4. Is the patient likely to manage the opioid therapy responsibly (or relevant caregiver likely to responsibly comanage)?

II.

1. Am I able to treat this patient without help?
2. Do I need the help of a pain specialist or other consultant to comanage this patient?
3. Are there appropriate specialists and resources available to help me comanage this patient?
4. Are the patient's medical, behavioral, or social circumstances so complex as to warrant referral to a pain medicine specialist for treatment?

Various sources, including published guidelines and statements from state medical boards, are available to help clinicians assess and monitor patients with persistent pain for responsible opioid use.

The recommendations also discussed the use of adjuvants. Adjuvants are agents developed for an indication other than pain that were later discovered to provide analgesia. This class includes antidepressants, anticonvulsants, and other agents that target neuronal cell surface proteins, such as ion channels and receptors. Based on high-quality evidence, the AGS guidelines give a strong recommendation that patients with neuropathic pain are candidates for treatment with adjuvant analgesics. Fibromyalgia also was noted as a consideration for a trial of an approved adjuvant medication. Lesser evidence supports trying adjuvant analgesics for other types of refractory persistent pain, such as back pain, headache, diffuse bone pain, and temporomandibular disorder.

Another concept that was discussed was that of using lower doses of multiple analgesics/adjuvants from different classes in a synergistic fashion to provide better pain relief than might be achieved by simply increasing the dose of a single agent. With this in mind, it is worth noting that the AGS strongly recommends that tertiary tricyclic antidepressants, including amitriptyline, imipramine, and doxepin, should be avoided in older adults due to their high risk for adverse consequences: anticholinergic effects and cognitive impairment. Also, the consensus recommendations from a geriatric clinical pharmacist expert panel were to reduce the dose of gabapentin when prescribed for pain in patients with renal dysfunction [3]. Specifically, patients with a creatinine clearance of 30–59 mL/min should have a maximum dose of 600 mg twice daily, 15–29 mL/min limited to 300 mg twice daily, and <15 mL/min prescribed no more than 300 mg per day [3].

Other options beyond traditional analgesics for treating persistent pain are considered less reliable according to the most recent AGS guidelines [1]. These include corticosteroids, muscle relaxants, benzodiazepines, calcitonin, bisphosphonates, and topical analgesics. Because of the low-quality evidence available, many nontraditional agents, such as glucosamine, chondroitin, cannabinoids, botulinum toxin, alpha-2 adrenergic agonists, calcitonin, vitamin D, bisphosphonates, and ketamine may be considered, but due to lack of research, some will need great caution in older subjects until data establishes their safety and efficacy. Additionally, the AGS strongly recommends that long-term systemic corticosteroids should only be used in older adults to treat pain-associated inflammatory disorders or metastatic bone pain due to substantial risk for adverse events established.

The AGS guidelines strongly support the use of topical lidocaine for treating localized neuropathic pain, and the analgesic is also weakly recommended for localized nonneuropathic pain. The other topical agents with recommendations, although weak, are topical NSAIDs for treatment of localized nonneuropathic persistent pain, and capsaicin or menthol for regional pain syndromes.

For muscle spasms recommendations are limited. Muscle relaxant drugs include cyclobenzaprine, carisoprodol, chlorzoxazone, methocabamol, and others. Readers should be aware that cyclobenzaprine is a drug that is essentially identical to amitriptyline with potential adverse effects similar to amitriptyline. Additionally, carisoprodol has been removed from the European market due to concerns about drug abuse. Although these drugs may relieve skeletal muscle pain, their effects are nonspecific and not related to muscle relaxation [4]. Therefore, these drugs should not be prescribed in the mistaken belief that they relieve muscle spasm. Muscle relaxants may inhibit polysynaptic myogenic reflexes in animal models, but whether this is related to pain relief remains unknown. If muscle spasm is suspected to be at the root of the patient's pain, it is probably justified to consider another drug with known effects on muscle spasm (e.g., benzodiazepines and baclofen).

Baclofen is an agonist of the gamma amino butyric acid type B (GABAB). Although its efficacy has been documented as a second-line drug for paroxysmal neuropathic pain, it has been utilized for patients with severe spasticity as a result of central nervous system injury, demyelinating conditions, and other neuromuscular disorders [5]. The common side effects of dizziness, somnolence, and gastrointestinal symptoms may be minimized by starting with a low dose and gradually increasing the prescribed amount. Discontinuation following prolonged use requires a slow tapering period because of the potential for delirium and seizure.

Summary

While acetaminophen remains the first-line recommendation by the AGS among the nonopioid class, it is recognized that most patients who visit the health care professional will have already tried this intervention. NSAIDs are discouraged in older adults for long-term use. If needed, a topical formulation can be prescribed or perhaps, oral naproxen can be co-prescribed along with an agent for gastrointestinal protection. Opioids are indeed acceptable for older adults. Despite the population's low risk for addiction, proper precautions should always be implemented when prescribing opioids. The Federation of State Medical Boards and other sources provide guidance for the appropriate prescribing practices and documentation necessary for managing patients with opioids. Constipation remains a concern for older adults on opioids. Methylnaltrexone is now an option for opioid-induced constipation.

Regularly scheduled dosing is recommended for patients with persistent pain, particularly those with cognitive impairment who are unable to vocalize their need for analgesia. Regular reassessments with instruments standardized in similar populations as the individual being treated should be conducted to ensure ongoing pain control and alternative therapies, such as physical therapy, cognitive behavioral therapy, and patient/caregiver education, should be combined with pharmacotherapies in order to optimize functional gains in older patients with persistent pain. Ideally pharmacotherapies that are selected will treat multiple issues (such as depression and pain) and reflect safety with regard to other comorbid conditions that a patient may have. Combination pharmacotherapeutic approaches that use complementary mechanistic actions or synergism for enhanced effects may optimize pain relief while limiting adverse events in patients who have dose-limiting adverse effects.

References

1. AGS Panel on Chronic Pain in Older Persons. The management of chronic pain in older persons. American Geriatrics Society. J Am Geriatr Soc. 1998;46:635–51.
2. American Geriatrics Society Panel on the Pharmacological Management of Persistent Pain in Older Persons. Pharmacological management of persistent pain in older persons. J Am Geriatr Soc. 2009;57(8):1331–46.
3. Hanlon JT, Aspinall SL, Semla TP, Weisbord SD, Fried LF, Good CB, et al. Consensus guidelines for oral dosing of primarily renally cleared medications in older adults. J Am Geriatr Soc. 2009;57(2):335–40.
4. Lussier D, Portenoy RK. Adjuvant analgesics in pain management. In: Douyle D, Hanks G, Cherny N, Calman K, editors. Oxford textbook of palliative medicine. 3rd ed. New York, NY: Oxford University Press; 2004. p. 349–78.
5. Fromm GH. Baclofen as an adjuvant analgesic. J Pain Symptom Manage. 1994;9:500–9.

Chapter 5
Spirituality as an Adjunct to Pain Management

Cristina Rosca Sichitiu and Thomas Mulligan

> *Nothing in life is more wonderful than Faith – the one great moving force which we can neither weigh in the balance nor test in the crucible.*
>
> Sir William Osler

Pain as a Complex, Multidimensional Experience

Thirty years ago George L. Engel [1] highlighted the limitations of the traditional biomedical model and advocated the endorsement of a biopsychosocial model. The application of the biopsychosocial framework to the management of the different aspects of disease facilitates understanding of the bidirectional influence between biological factors on the one hand and psychological, social, and spiritual factors on the other hand.

In the biopsychosocial model, pain comprises four distinct components: physical (the perception of physical pain), emotional (the anxiety, depression, or psychological distress associated with pain), social (the isolation and abandonment often associated with pain), and spiritual (the agonizing search for meaning – why me). Further research on the multidimensional aspects of pain gave shape to new theoretical models like the Gate Control Theory and the Neuromatrix Theory [2, 3] that emphasize the role of psychological factors as mediators for pain.

More recently, there has been a call for a biopsychosocial-spiritual framework. According to this model, every patient has a spiritual history that helps shape who each patient is as a whole. Major efforts are being made to try to delineate valid measurement tools for the relationship to an immeasurable domain – the transcendent. Four measurement domains of spirituality in health care are proposed: religiosity

T. Mulligan (✉)
Medical director Senior Services, St. Bernards Health Care, Jonesboro, AR, USA
e-mail: tmulligan@sbrmc.org

F.M. Gloth, III (ed.), *Handbook of Pain Relief in Older Adults: An Evidence-Based Approach*, Aging Medicine, DOI 10.1007/978-1-60761-618-4_5,
© Springer Science+Business Media, LLC 2011

(strength of belief, prayer, and worship practices), spiritual (coping, response to disease in terms of spiritual attitudes and practices), spiritual well-being (level of spiritual distress), and spiritual needs (conversation, prayer, ritual) [4].

The Spiritual Dimension of Disease

The spiritual dimension is an integral component of most people. Although spirituality is subjective, and difficult to define or measure, several researchers took upon themselves the challenge of exploring this aspect of patient care from an evidence-based perspective.

The vast majority (95%) of Americans reports a belief in God, and almost 75% claim that their view of life is determined by their religious beliefs [5]. Among older Americans, 98% believe in God and 95% pray regularly [6].

Extant studies show that nearly 80% of adults in the USA believe that religion helps patients and families cope with illness [7]. About 75% of the public believes that praying for someone can help cure his or her illness, and 56% state that faith has helped them recover from illness, injury, or disease [8]. American adults also consistently state that they welcome a discussion with their physicians about spirituality: 83% of patients surveyed in Ohio report that they want physicians to ask about spiritual beliefs, especially during serious illness [9].

In response to the importance of spirituality in medical decisions and its impact on health and quality of life, the Joint Commission for the Accreditation of Healthcare Organizations (JCAHO) now requires that patient spirituality be addressed as part of routine inpatient care as well as part of the palliative services [10]. Despite patient's interest and need, a nationwide survey of 1,732,562 patients report low rates of satisfaction with the spiritual care they receive [11].

When pain occurs, patients typically seek relief, often resorting to spirituality. For example, in a study of hospitalized patients experiencing pain, spiritual activity was used almost as often as analgesics (62% vs. 67%, respectively [12]. But, does spiritual activity really help? Thus far, at least 34 studies have assessed the relationship between spirituality and health outcomes, almost all of which reported a beneficial effect [13]. In addition, ten studies have specifically evaluated the relationship between spirituality and pain. Three of these (one randomized controlled trial) found that spirituality was associated with alleviation of pain [14].

Although data are still sparse, pain seems to diminish in response to spiritual activity. Serotonin receptor density in the brain may be related to spiritual proclivities. This finding opens up the possibility that spiritual practices may influence serotonin pathways in the brain that may regulate pain perception [15].

Does spirituality still help as hope for a cure diminishes? For example, does prayer help the terminal patient? Spirituality is often used as a coping strategy by patients with incurable diseases. For example, among patients admitted to a nursing home, 86% used spirituality (e.g., prayer, Bible reading) as a means to cope with declining health [16]. Use of spirituality in patients who are nearing death probably helps because spiritual activity is associated with an improved mood, thereby [17] providing hope (the hope of an afterlife, hope of seeing loved ones again in heaven) [18].

Relationship Between Physical and Spiritual Pain

The recognition of the complex emotional and spiritual aspects of pain finds its expression in the definition of suffering as "the state of severe distress associated with events that threaten the intactness of the person" [19]. Dame Cicely Saunders identified meaninglessness as "the essence of spiritual pain" [20].

On the one hand, physical pain can contribute to spiritual pain by challenging one's sense of meaning and hope. Pain may challenge a person's assumptions about the world (e.g., I will live a long and happy life). Once these assumptions or models are proven inadequate, a person will look for new satisfactory models and explanations in a quest for new meanings. Several interpretations of pain from a spiritual perspective have been proposed [21]. Listed below are a few examples with some of the possible spiritual perspectives.

Interpretations of Personal Suffering

Theodical Theory	Example
Punishment	My pain is the result of my sins
Testing	God is testing my loyalty to Him
Resignation to God's Will	God willed it, I don't understand it
Redemption	I understand Christ's suffering

Adapted from [21]

On the other hand, spiritual health can influence pain perception and the patient's coping mechanisms. An analysis of the use of positive and negative religious coping in patients suffering from chronic pain was one of the first studies to provide evidence that positive religious coping has unique effects on adjustment to pain beyond what can be explained on the basis of demographics and pain level. For some patients, the main spiritual theme consisted of a positive frame where one looks to a higher power for strength, comfort, and support. Positive religious coping tended to be adaptive. Negative religious coping consisted of two main subtypes: patients with the "Punishing God" view saw the pain as retribution from God, and patients with the "Absent God" view felt abandoned by God during the time when they most needed support. Beyond exploring the two aspects of the relationship between pain and spirituality, one of the most crucial findings of this study was that positive forms of religious coping were related to significantly higher levels of positive affect and more positive spiritual and religious outcomes [22].

One of the most systematic studies recently published showed how positive and negative forms of religious coping affect adjustment to persistent pain. This study found that positive religious coping techniques were related to significantly better mental health, while negative religious coping (i.e., feeling punished or abandoned by God) was related to significantly poorer physical and mental health outcomes [23].

As there is growing interest in the possibility that interventions that encourage positive religious coping might be beneficial in managing pain, several other studies were conducted. A 30-day diary study found that rheumatoid arthritis patients who reported positive religious and spiritual coping strategies were better able to control their pain; they experienced much lower levels of pain and negative mood, as well as much higher levels of social support. These findings suggest that spiritual coping variables are meaningfully related to the experience of chronic arthritis pain [24].

Another recent study found that by using spiritual meditation at least 20 min a day, patients with frequent migraine headaches were able to improve their pain tolerance and reduce headache frequency and severity. Those regularly practicing spiritual meditation also experienced improvements in mental, physical, and spiritual health. These findings show that patients with chronic pain conditions can be taught to use their spiritual resources in order to reduce the negative impact of pain [25].

Cultural Issues and Spirituality

Spirituality and religion are not the same but are overlapping concepts. Spirituality can be defined as a belief framework that gives meaning and sense of wholeness to life [26]. This is usually expressed as religion or relationship with God. The word religion is derived from the Latin religare meaning "to bind together." It is a structured belief system that addresses spiritual questions and provides a framework for making sense of day to day life [27].

Virtually all cultures provide explanatory models that attempt to account for infirmities and sufferings in the life of a human being. Religion and spirituality are among the most important cultural factors that give meaning and purpose to one's existence [28]. Meeting our patient's needs in a multi-cultural society is challenging but important. The patient's culture influences the perception of illness and its treatment options.

The three monotheistic religions, Judaism, Christianity, and Islam, believe in the same God, the God of Abraham, hence the common designation as the "Abrahamic" religions. However, observance of traditional beliefs and practices varies within each of these religions. And, each of these three religious groups typically has denominations or sub-groups.

In Judaism, religion and culture are intertwined. Judaism is based on the worship of the God of Abraham, with the Jewish law based on the Old Testament of the Bible (written law) and the Talmud (oral law). Judaism is integral to the life of religiously observant Jews, and even secular Jewish patients often welcome the wisdom of their tradition when considering treatment options. Traditional or religious Jews typically have concerns about modesty in the health-care setting, and many appreciate being cared for by nurses or physicians of the same sex [29]. Illness is interpreted in the context of their religious perspective, and religion is used as a source of meaning and hope in times of illness [30].

The Christian believes in the God of Abraham but also believes that God has three distinct beings (God the Father, Jesus the Christ, and the Holy Spirit), based on the Old and New Testaments of the Bible. They believe that every person has been made in the image of God but has been tainted by the sin of Adam. Jesus' death on the cross provides atonement for the sinful nature of those who place their faith in Jesus. It is this faith in Jesus that transforms them into Christians (forgiven sinners) [31]. Illness can be perceived as punishment from God (for sin), refinement (strengthening through trials), or the incomprehensible will of the omniscient God who can be trusted in all things [30].

Among American Christians, Mexican Americans are predominantly Roman Catholic, and demonstrate an association between church attendance and life satisfaction [32]. Mexican Americans also exhibit a strong emphasis on prayer as a coping mechanism [32]. Similarly, African Americans are often deeply religious. More than 90% of older adults use religion to cope with the stress of medical problems, with African American women using religious coping more often than non-African American women [33]. However, there is great diversity of religious beliefs and practices in African Americans. Some are Catholics, there is a growing number of Muslims, but the majority is evangelical Christian. Thus, religion plays a major role in the lives of most African Americans who rely on the comfort, hope, and meaning it provides [34].

Islam worships God as Allah and reveres the prophet Muhammad. The Muslim framework of values is linked to the Qur'an and the tradition of the Prophet Muhammad. To the Muslim, God is the ultimate healer. Islam teaches that the patient must be treated with respect and compassion, and that the physical, mental, and spiritual dimensions of the illness be taken into account. Many Muslims invoke the name of God in daily conversation, pray five times a day facing Mecca, and wash prior to prayer. They believe that their actions are accountable and subject to ultimate judgment [35].

In the Native American population, healing, spirituality, and culture are closely intertwined. Intuition and spiritual awareness are a healer's most essential diagnostic tools. Therapeutic methods include prayer, ceremonies, music, herbalism, and massage. Participation of family and friends is a large component of these healing interventions [36]. Native American healing is based on wholeness, balance, harmony, and meaning [37]. Understanding the various spiritual/religious and cultural issues involved for the individual patient assists the health-care provider in delivering a more efficient and compassionate care.

Hindus and Sikhs, though their cultural and religious traditions have differences, share a belief in rebirth, a concept of karma, an emphasis on purity, and a view of the person that affirms family, culture, environment, and the spiritual dimension [38].

Traditional Chinese medicine views the body and spirit as an integrated whole. This perspective is influenced primarily by Confucianism but also by Taoism and Buddhism. Illness is believed to be a result of an imbalance of a vital energy force called QI and Ying/Yang Bowman [39]. Mankind and nature are considered interdependent; harmony of this nature–human relationship is vital to health [40].

Clinical Goals of Spiritual Assessment and Care

The following is a spiritual-care strategy proposed by Plotnikoff in Rakel's *Integrative Medicine* [41]. Five goals of the spiritual assessment are identified as follows:

- *Goal 1: Anticipate the presence of religious and spiritual concerns.* Health-care professionals should be aware that any medical situation can represent a moment of crisis, and that religious and spiritual concerns can be implicit and unconscious both to the patient and to the physician. Being prepared to attentively listen to patient concerns without judgment can be both a diagnostic and a therapeutic tool.
- *Goal 2: Comprehend how patients want their religious and spiritual beliefs to be seen as resources for strength.* Since every religion has teachings and rituals that may be unknown to the health-care provider, physicians should be prepared to allow the patient to clarify what is important.
- *Goal 3: Understand your patients' experiences and perception of the transcendent.* Since many health-care professionals are familiar with only a small number of religious worldviews, they are at risk of extrapolating from one patient's cultural group and making it the truth for all such patients. The clinician should be careful to individualize his understanding of what a particular illness means for an individual patient.
- *Goal 4: Determine what impact, positive or negative, your patients' spiritual orientation has on their health problems and perceived needs.* Spiritual suffering can result from the loss of the patient's physical, social, and spiritual connections: betrayal by one's body, loss of social role, or theological doubt. Restoring hope and meaning to a suffering person may be a challenging task as this consists of identifying what is important for the patient and trying to help him/her achieve his/her goals.
- *Goal 5: Determine appropriate referrals to chaplains, clergy, or traditional healers for spiritual care.* The clinician's role in spiritual care is supportive and respectful. The questions asked are there to help the patient find answers in a spiritual quest. Where chaplains trained in Clinical Pastoral Education (CPE) are available, they should be asked for their assistance in responding to spiritual concerns.

Practical Application

Outlined below are three methods and mnemonics for spiritual assessment that can guide physicians in their interview. They provide questions that may lead to valuable insights on care for the patient. The information gathered from a spiritual history often reveals the importance of spirituality to the patient and guides health-care professionals in how we can offer support, especially in times of medical crisis.

SPIRIT [42]	
S	*Spiritual* belief system – What is your religious affiliation?
P	*Personal spirituality* – Describe the beliefs and practices of your religion or spiritual system that you personally accept/do not accept
I	*Integration* within a spiritual community – Do you belong to a spiritual or religious group or community?
R	*Ritualized* practices and restrictions – Are there specific practices that you carry out as part of your religion/spirituality? What significance do these practices or restrictions have to you?
I	*Implications* for medical care – What aspects of your religion/spirituality would you like me to keep in mind as I care for you?
T	*Terminal* events planning – As we plan for your care near the end of life, how does your faith impact your decisions?

HOPE [43]	
H	*Hope* – What are your sources of hope, meaning, strength, peace, love, and connectedness?
O	*Organization* – Do you consider yourself part of an organized religion?
P	*Personal* spirituality and practices – What aspects of your spirituality or spiritual practices do you find most helpful?
E	*Effects* – How do your beliefs affect the kind of medical care you would like me to provide?

FICA [44]	
F	*Faith* or belief – What is your faith or belief?
I	*Importance* – Is it important in your life? How?
C	*Community* – Are you part of a religious community?
A	*Addressing* – What would you want me as your physician to be aware of? How would you like me to address these issues in your care?

Thus, interventions to relieve pain should make use of spirituality. The basic goal of attending to spirituality in pain management is to help strengthen patients' resources so they can better cope. By exploring potential spiritual meanings of pain, the health-care provider can gain a better understanding of a patient's perception of pain and thus provide more effective and satisfactory care [45].

An empathetic exploration of patient's pain can also identify the possibility of spiritual pain as hopelessness and lack of meaning. Health-care providers can assist patients by reframing expectations, thus offering hope in a new context. Psychiatrists, Frankl and Yalom [46], suggested methods by which meaning can be created and hope restored.

Meaning Restoration Strategies

Strategy	Explanation
Altruism	Leaving the world a better place
Dedication to a cause	Religious, political, or social
Creativity	Generating something new
Hedonism	Appreciating remaining life to the fullest
Self-actualization	Developing one's full potential
Self-transcendence	Placing one's focus away from self

If the patient is religious, the clinician may offer to pray with him or her. Intercessory prayer, as an adjunct to standard treatment for pain, is beneficial [47]. Prayer is facilitated when both patient and physician are of the same faith (e.g., Jewish, Christian, etc.). When the patient and physician have differing beliefs, the physician must be respectful of the patient's faith. This approach has the advantage of fostering the patient–doctor therapeutic relationship. Short prayers that focus on healing and relief of pain are often helpful. Devotional practices, such as reading the Bible, Bhagavad Gita, and Qur'an may also be helpful. If the patient is religious but the health-care professional is unable or prefers not to engage in prayer or discussions of a religious nature, he/she should request the assistance of a chaplain or the patient's own religious leader (e.g., pastor, rabbi, priest, etc).

In conclusion, many people believe that we are spiritual beings with needs that contribute to pain or its alleviation. When health-care providers incorporate the spiritual aspect of the patient into the care provided, they often gain better insight into the patient's perceptions and are more successful at relieving pain.

References

1. Engel GL. The need for a new medical model: a challenge for biomedicine. Science. 1977;196:129–36.
2. Melzack R. From the gate to the neuromatrix. Pain. 1999;S6:S121–26.
3. Wacholtz AB, Pearce MJ. Exploring the relationship between spirituality, coping and pain. J Behav Med. 2007;30:311–18.
4. Sulmasy DP. A biopsychosocial-spiritual model for the care of patients at the end of life. Gerontologist. 2002;42:24–33.

5. Gallup G. Religion in America. Princeton: Religious Research Center; 1990.
6. Koenig HG. Religious behaviors and death anxiety in later life. Hospice J. 1988;4:3–24.
7. Dujardin RC. Faith in medicine. Detroit Free Press. 26 Dec 1996;7D
8. McNichol T: When religion and medicine meet: the new faith in medicine. USA Weekend. 7 April 1996;4.
9. McCord G, Gilchrist VJ, Grossman SD, King BD, McCormick KE, Oprandi AM, et al. Discussing spirituality with patients: a rational and ethical approach. Ann Fam Med. 2004;2:356–61.
10. Joint Commission on Accreditation of Healthcare Organizations. Comprehensive accreditation manual for hospitals. Oakbrook Terrace: Joint Commission on Accreditation of Healthcare Organizations; 2003. http://www.pohly.com/books/comprehensiveaccreditation-hospitals.html
11. Clark PA, Drain M, Malone MP. Addressing patient's emotional and spiritual needs. Jt Comm J Qual Saf. 2003;29:659–70.
12. McNaill JA, Sherwood GA, Starck PL, Thompson CJ. Assessing clinical outcomes: patient satisfaction with pain management. J Pain Symptom Manage. 1998;16:29–40.
13. Townsend M, Ayele H, Mulligan T. Systematic review of clinical trials examining the effects of religion on health. South Med Assoc J. 2002;95:1429–34.
14. Koenig HG. Religion and medicine IV: religion, physical health, and clinical implications. Int J Psychiatry Med. 2001;31:321–36.
15. Borg J, Andree B, Soderstrom H, Farde L. The serotonin system and spiritual experiences. Am J Psychiatry. 2003;160:1965–69.
16. Ayele H, Mulligan T, Gheorghiu S, Reyes-Ortiz C. Religious activity improves life satisfaction for some physicians and older patients. J Am Geriatr Soc. 1999;47:453–5.
17. Musick M, Koening, H, Hays, J, Cohen H. Religious activity and depression among community-dwelling elderly persons with cancer: the moderating effect of race. J Gerontol B Psychol Sci Soc Sci. 1998;53B:S218–27.
18. Newshan G. Transcending the physical: spiritual aspects of pain in patients with HIV and/or cancer. J Adv Nurs. 1998;28:1236–41.
19. Cassel EJ. The nature of suffering and the goals of medicine. N Engl J Med. 1982;306:639–645.
20. Saunders C. Spiritual pain. J Palliat Care. 1988;4(3):29–32.
21. Foley DP. Eleven interpretations of personal suffering. J Relig Health. 1988;27:321–8.
22. Bush EG, Rye MS, Brant CR, Emery E, Pargament KI, Riessinger CA. Religious coping with chronic pain. Appl Psychophysiol Biofeedback. 1999;24:249–60.
23. Rippentrop EA, Altmaier EM, Chen JJ, Found EM, Keffala VJ. The relationship between religion/spirituality and physical health, mental health, and pain in a chronic pain population. Pain. 2005;116:311–21.
24. Keefe FJ, Affleck G, Lefebvre J, Underwood L, Caldwell DS, Drew J. Living with rheumatoid arthritis: the role of daily spirituality and daily religious and spiritual coping. J Pain 2001;2:101–10.
25. Wachholtz AB. Does spirituality matter? Effects of meditative content and orientation on migraineurs [doctoral dissertation]. Bowling Green: Bowling Green State University, 2006. Available from: http://www.ohiolink.edu/etd/view.cgi?bgsu1143662175 accessed 14 Jul 2009.
26. McBride JL, Arthur G, Brooks R, Pilkington L. The relationship between a patient's spirituality and health experiences. Fam Med. 1998;30:122–6.
27. Webster's encyclopedic unabridged dictionary of the English language. New York: Portland House; 1996.
28. O'Brien M. Integrative geriatrics: combining traditional and alternative medicine. N C Med J. 1996;57:364–7.
29. Goldsand G, Rosenberg Z, Gordonv M. Bioethics for clinicians: 22. Jewish bioethics. CMAJ. 2001;164:219–22.
30. Kappelli S. Between suffering and redemption. Religious motives in Jewish and Christian cancer patients' coping. Scand J Caring Sci. 2000;14:82–8.

31. Pauls M, Hutchinson R. Bioethics for clinicians: 28. Protestant bioethics. CMAJ. 2002;166:339–43.
32. Gelfand D, Balcazar H, Parzuchowski J, Lenox S. Mexicans and care for the terminally ill: family, hospice, and the church. Am J Hosp Palliat Care. 2001;18:391–6.
33. Conway K. Coping with the stress of medical problems among black and white elderly. Int J Aging Hum Dev. 1985;21:39–48.
34. Levin JS, Chatters LM, Taylor RJ. Religious effects on health status and life satisfaction among black Americans. J Gerontol B Psychol Sci Soc Sci. 1995;50B:S154–63.
35. Sarhill N, LeGrand S, Islamabouli BS, Davis MP, Walsh D. The terminally ill Muslim: death and dying from the Muslim perspective. Am J Hosp Palliat Care. 2001;18:251–5.
36. Kim C, Kwok Y. Navajo use of native healers. Arch Int Med. 1998;158:2245–9.
37. Weigand DA. Traditional Native American medicine in dermatology. Clin Dermatol. 1999;17:49–51.
38. Coward H, Sidhu T. Bioethics for clinicians: 19. Hinduism and Sikhism. CMAJ. 2000;163:1167–70.
39. Bowman KW, Hui EC. Bioethics for clinicians: 20. Chinese bioethics. CMAJ. 2000;163:1481–5.
40. Zhang J, Verhoef MJ. Illness management strategies among Chinese immigrants living with arthritis. Soc Sci Med. 2002;55:1795–1802.
41. Plotnikoff GA. Rakel: integrative medicine, 2nd ed., 2007; Sect. 8, Chap. 112.
42. Maugans TA. The SPIRITual history. Arch Fam Med. 1996;5:11–6.
43. Anandarajah G, Hight E. Spirituality and medical practice: using the HOPE questions as a practical tool for spiritual assessment. Am Fam Phys. 2001;63:81–8.
44. Puchalski CM, Larsen DB, Post SG. Physicians and patient spirituality. Ann Intern Med. 2000;133:748–9.
45. McGuire D, Henke Yarboro C. Cancer pain management. Philadelphia: Saunders; 1995. Chap. 3, p. 52.
46. Yalom ID. Existential psychotherapy. New York: Basic Books; 1980.
47. Matthews D, Marlowe S, MacNutt F. Effects of intercessory prayer on patients with rheumatoid arthritis. South Med J. 2009;93:1177–86.

Chapter 6
The Role of Rehabilitation in Managing Pain in Seniors

Mark J. Gloth and Richard A. Black

> *Lack of activity destroys the good condition of every human being, while movement and methodical physical exercise save it and preserve it.*

> Plato

Since Plato first spoke those words, physical medicine and rehabilitation have played an increasingly important and well-substantiated role in the management of pain in the elderly. The basic principles of rehabilitation in the geriatric population are to prevent disability, treat specific impairments, prevent secondary disability, restore functional ability, and prevent handicaps by adapting to disability. To fully understand these principles, the progression of pain must be understood from a rehabilitation perspective. Pain as an impairment is the loss or abnormality of a psychological, physiologic, or anatomic structure or function. Pain is defined as a disability when the impairment restricts a person's ability to perform a task or activity within the normal range of human ability. Pain as a disability then becomes a handicap when it causes enough of a disadvantage that it interferes with a person's ability to interact with the environment.

This progression often is the result of what is described as the vicious cycle of pain. Pain triggers muscle tension. Positioning to avoid pain leads to strain on some muscles and disuse of others. Unused muscles lose strength, causing inflammation, swelling, and stiffness. Inflamed tissues cause compression between the skin and muscle, resulting in constriction of lymphatic fluid flow. This compression causes pressure to the pain receptors below the skin. This results in signals to the brain that increase stress and the release of fight-or-flight chemicals (i.e., norepinephrine) and the restriction of neurotransmitters like serotonin, resulting in mental and physical fatigue and depression. Hence, the vicious cycle of pain continues.

Although there are a large variety of widely accepted therapeutic modalities for treating this vicious cycle of pain, the multifactorial issues that contribute to pain

M.J. Gloth (✉)
HCR ManorCare, 333 N. Summit Street, Toledo, Ohio 43699-0086
e-mail: magloth@hcr-manorcare.com

F.M. Gloth, III (ed.), *Handbook of Pain Relief in Older Adults: An Evidence-Based Approach*, Aging Medicine, DOI 10.1007/978-1-60761-618-4_6,
© Springer Science+Business Media, LLC 2011

in the elderly, combined with numerous methodic problems, demand an interdisciplinary treatment approach. Exercise and physical modalities should be at the core of this approach to managing pain in the geriatric patient.

Exercise

Physical activity has been recognized as an important aspect of patient care for nearly 50 years [1] and has been shown to improve pain significantly in older patients [1]. Bortz's "disuse syndrome" suggests that physical inactivity can predictably lead to deterioration of multiple body and organ-specific functions [2]. Physiological changes such as osteoporosis, degenerative joint disease, obesity, and muscle atrophy, which may contribute to pain syndromes, are combated with exercise. In fact, immobility and bed rest longer than 2 days have never been shown to be beneficial and, on the contrary, appear to be detrimental in the geriatric patient population [1].

Clinical trials involving older patients with chronic musculoskeletal pain have shown that moderate levels of training on a regular basis are effective in improving pain and functional status [3]. Training in the form of endurance exercises, strengthening programs, and the martial arts has been demonstrated to prevent the physiological changes associated with pain.

Endurance training includes aerobic activities such as walking, jogging, running, cycling, and swimming. Regular aerobic exercise is generally believed to raise the pain threshold by stimulating the release of endogenous opioids [4]. In addition, the weight loss associated with these activities has been shown to reduce the severity of joint pain significantly. Swimming and pool exercises cause less joint stress and, when done in a heated pool, may actually provide analgesia. For an aerobic exercise program to be effective, however, it must be well tolerated. The activity must use large muscle groups, incorporate repetitive muscle contractions, and elevate the resting heart rate to the target heart rate for at least 20 min [5]. Target intensity in the geriatric patient has been effective at 40% of maximum [5].

The exercise prescription should include the warm-up, the conditioning period, and the cool down. Specifications should include activity, frequency, duration, intensity, and precautions. Of course, exercise with an acutely inflamed or significantly swollen joint should be deferred until the inflammation has subsided.

Strength training may also have significant protective benefits in the prevention of pain. Strength training may occur with the use of free weights, elastic exercise bands, or other resistive exercise equipment. Patients in their 90s have shown significant gains in muscle strength, size, and functional mobility [6]. Progressive resistive exercises have been responsible for marked improvements in pain management and functional ability [7–9]. Caution must be used with isometric exercise (i.e., muscle contractions without joint movement). Although this form of exercise is particularly useful in providing improved endurance and tone without stressing joints, it may transiently increase the blood pressure by as much as 20 mmHg with sustained contractions.

Initial training usually requires 8–12 weeks of supervision by a knowledgeable professional who can focus on the specific needs of older adults with musculoskeletal conditions. Best results are realized when the program is maintained indefinitely to prevent deconditioning and deterioration. Although the role of a structured therapeutic exercise program in the treatment of acute low back pain may be questioned, several authors noted that exercise programs promote flexibility, strength, and generalized conditioning, which play a significant role in pain management [10–11]. Activity alone may play a preventive role in pain simply by preventing the physiological changes that occur to produce pains.

Tai chi, with its focus on breathing and flowing gestures, is often described as "meditation in motion" [12]. It emerged sometime between the 1300s and the 1600s in China. Some say it was developed by monks, others by a retired general. They agree its ancient roots are in the martial arts, but tai chi movements are never aggressive. They are based on shifting body weight through a series of light, controlled movements that flow rhythmically into one long, graceful gesture. The sequences have poetic names, such as "waving hand in the cloud" or "pushing the mountain," and can be quite beautiful to an observer [13].

Although there are no good, controlled studies that proved tai chi specifically benefits people with arthritis by reducing pain or inflammation, there is a study from 1991 that evaluated its safety for patients with rheumatoid arthritis [14]. It concluded that 10 weeks of tai chi classes did not make joint problems worse and said the weight-bearing aspects of this exercise have the potential to stimulate bone growth and strengthen connective tissue.

It is widely thought that mind–body alternatives, such as tai chi and meditation, that focus on psychological as well as physical function could be beneficial when used with conventional medications. However, scientific investigation of the therapeutic values of tai chi is still lacking.

Physical Agent Modalities

Physical Agent Modalities for pain management have been used for many years as nonpharmacological interventions for pain management. Although there have been many studies demonstrating positive physiological effects of modalities on biologic tissues [15–20], other studies often have conflicting results [21–23]. Most reviews agree, however, that there is a need for additional well-designed studies in order to better understand the effectiveness of physical modalities. Nonetheless, when modalities are carefully selected based on the patient's condition, the goals of treatment, indications and contraindications for treatment; they can be a safe, effective means of progressing toward the patient's treatment goals. Physical Agent Modalities should act as an adjunct to a comprehensive nonpharmacological treatment plan for addressing pain rather than an isolated treatment approach.

Heat vs. Cold

The debate over heat and cold is as old as the modalities themselves. The advantage of cryotherapy appears to be in its rapid analgesic effect, reduction of acute inflammation, and prevention of edema in the acute injury. Thermal therapy allows increased tissue extensibility and relaxation. This would suggest that cold followed by heat would allow the most efficacious and synergistic use of these modalities in pain management. Indeed, studies have suggested that superficial heat and cold as described in the following sections have similar positive effects on relieving pain, most likely because of their similar mechanisms of action [24–27].

Cryotherapy

Cryotherapy is defined as the use of cold modalities for treatment purposes. This superficial means of cooling is known to have a local analgesic effect and to reduce inflammatory responses and muscle spasms [28]. The analgesic effect arises from a combination of altered neural transmission, reduced muscle spasm, altered blood flow to muscle and nerve, and increased endorphin production [28]. There is no indication, however, that a particular type of cold application consistently is more effective than another. Cryotherapy is most commonly used for the initial management of such acute musculoskeletal and soft tissue injuries as sprains and strains, for spasticity management, to treat myofascial pain syndrome, and for postoperative pain treatment. Chronic conditions treated with cryotherapy include tendonitis, bursitis, trigger points, and muscle spasm. Types of cryotherapy include cold packs (−12°F), chemical gel packs, ice packs (cools 5°C at 2-cm depth), ice massage, vapocoolant sprays, controlled cold-compression units, and cold water immersion (4–10°C for 30 s).

Thermal Therapy

In physical medicine, locally applied heat agents are used not only to promote relaxation and pain relief, but also to increase blood flow, facilitate tissue healing, and prepare stiff joints and tight muscles for exercise. The physiological effects of heat are analgesia, increased metabolism, muscle relaxation, and sedation. The temperature gradient theory described by Wells [29] in 1947 combined with other mechanisms (including the gate theory and the release of endorphins) that result from heating tissues provide the most likely explanation for increased analgesic effects. Heat produces increased metabolism by arteriolar dilation, causing increased capillary flow and pressure, which subsequently clear metabolites, speed chemical processes, and increase the supply of oxygen, leukocytes, antibodies, and nutrients. This in turn can cause acute edema but can subsequently clear chronic edema by the same mechanism. Muscle relaxation occurs from heating secondary to effects on local muscle spindle and Golgi tendon responses.

Therapeutic heat is indicated in a variety of painful conditions. Specific modalities of heat are categorized by mode of transfer and depth of heating. Primary modes of heat transfer are through conduction (hot packs and paraffin baths), convection (fluidotherapy and hydrotherapy), or conversion (radiant heat, laser, microwaves, short waves, or ultrasound).

Ultrasound is a mechanical vibration transmitted at a frequency above the upper limit of human hearing. It causes the molecules of biologic tissues to oscillate or vibrate and can be used therapeutically to accelerate wound healing. Ultrasound has thermal and nonthermal effects. Both the thermal and nonthermal effects are produced when the ultrasound is used in the continuous mode, whereas nonthermal effects are predominantly produced when the sound wave is periodically interrupted or "pulsed." While continuous ultrasound is more effective in increasing motor and sensory nerve conduction velocities allowing for pain reduction; pulsed ultrasound accelerated the inflammatory phases allowing for more rapid healing [30].

Phonophoresis is the use of ultrasound to enhance the transmission of medications through the skin to superficial tissues. Frequently, corticosteroids are mixed with ultrasound gel and the injured tissue is sonated. The advantage of this technique is that anti-inflammatory medications can be delivered directly to the affected tissue with a minimum amount entering the systemic circulation.

Monochromatic Red and Near-Infrared *Light Therapy* (IR) uses a single red (630–660 nm) and/or near Infra Red (880–890 nm) wavelength(s) of light emitted by super luminous diodes (SLDs) embedded in flexible rubber pads (SLD Light Therapy Pads) which are placed in close proximity to the patient's skin. The energy is absorbed by the skin and underlying tissues up to a depth of 5 cm dependent on the wavelength and tissue transmission. A variety of physiologic effects are associated with the absorption of monochromatic light in tissue including increased circulation, pain reduction, and stimulation of tissue repair.

Shortwave *Diathermy* heats body tissue by means of a high frequency oscillating electromagnetic field. It can be either continuous or pulsed. Continuous Shortwave Diathermy provides a constant output of electrical energy, whereas Pulsed Shortwave Diathermy simply interrupts the electromagnetic field at regular intervals to allow heat to dissipate and decrease the likelihood of any significant rise in tissue temperature.

Selecting the right heating modality is based on the principle of propagation and absorption [11]. The decision to use superficial vs. deep heat depends on the location of the involved structure and the temperature elevation desired. Deep heat is usually selected when tissue contracture exists, such as during the chronic phases after an injury or a disease [11]. Sensitivity to temperature and pain must be determined before making the decision to use superficial heat in a therapeutic regimen. Superficial heat should be used cautiously in patients with circulatory impairment and should probably not be used over any areas of arterial insufficiency. Deep heat is contraindicated in patients with a local malignancy or bleeding diathesis, with metal implants, and after laminectomy.

Risk of thermal injuries is increased in the geriatric patient if the patient is obtunded, has poor circulation, is sedated, or has impaired sensation. Therefore, particular care must be taken when writing a prescription for the use of thermal modalities. A prescription should include diagnosis, precautions, form of heat, intensity of heat, duration of therapy, and frequency of follow-up.

It is important to note that heat alone produces only short-term, immediate pain relief. When heat is combined with an exercise program, pain relief is greater and longer lasting, strength and function improve, and stiffness is reduced [11].

Electrotherapy

Electrotherapy stimulation is the use of electricity to obtain desired physiological responses for the care of muscle injuries. Melzack and Wall's description of a gating mechanism in the dorsal horn of the spinal cord [21] led to the development of numerous electrotherapy modalities, including conventional transcutaneous electrical nerve stimulation (TENS), acupuncture, noxious-level TENS, percutaneous electrical nerve stimulation, dorsal column stimulation, cranial electrical stimulation, interferential current therapy, pulsed electromagnetic therapy, and iontophoresis.

A change in neuronal activity is the most important physical effect elicited using electrical modalities of pain management. In addition to the segmented gating mechanisms, descending pain control systems or negative-feedback loops further modulate pain. Electrical stimulation of supraspinal brain stem sites also produce release of endorphins, which mediate pain by binding to opiate sites, thereby blocking pain transmission.

TENS has been widely accepted as an effective method of pain control for several chronic and acute conditions of the elderly. Unfortunately, there are few studies that disclose long-term, statistically significant evidence of improved function, decreased analgesic requirements, and shorter hospital stays. In a study of TENS in chronic low back pain, Deyo and co-workers [31] found that TENS provided no additional benefit to a home exercise program.

Pulsed electrical stimulation has been shown to improve pain, function, and stiffness [32, 33]. This device uses a capacitively coupled pulsed electrical stimulation device. This device is different from a TENS unit, in that it uses a monophasic spiked signal with a frequency of 100 Hz and voltage between 0–12 and is below the threshold of sensation [34]. The device attempts to mimic the electrical fields created in healthy articular cartilage [32].

Interferential electrical current (IFC) is a type of electrical stimulation commonly used to provide short-term relief of acute or chronic pain [35–38]. Interferential electrical stimulation uses two medium frequency sinusoidal carrier waves that are slightly out of phase and slightly different frequencies allowing the current to pass through the skin easily and then delivering a therapeutic low frequency wave to deep tissues. Contraindications would be the same as TENS and other forms of medium frequency-alternating current.

Iontophoresis is a form of electrical stimulation used for a variety of clinical issues. It involves the use of a very small direct current to drive medication into superficial tissue. Iontophoresis works on the principle that like charges repel each other. Iontophoresis also increases the permeability of the skin for peptide and protein molecules so that medications penetrate the skin more readily [39]. The site of injury must be relatively superficial so that the medication can reach it. There are a number of advantages and disadvantages to iontophoresis. The advantages are that there is a lower risk of infection since the skin is not broken, it is relatively painless compared to an injection, it avoids first-pass elimination by the liver, the drug delivery can be rapidly stopped by simply shutting down the device and removing the electrode with the medication on it and the medication can be delivered directly to the target tissue while minimizing the systemic effects [39]. The disadvantages are that it can only treat relatively superficial structures, drugs must be aqueous and ionized, other charged particles in the solution may compete with the drug of interest, the amount of medication that can be administered is limited and the skin itself acts as a barrier to the medication [39].

It is important to remember that electrotherapy involves the use of electricity on the body and hence follows principle precautions related to electricity and therefore precautions need to be carefully observed during treatment.

Manual Therapy

Traction and manual manipulation also may be effective in restoring motion and relieving pain. And, although there is no evidence in the current peer-reviewed literature to support these therapies, one would argue that there is case support for their effectiveness.

The purpose of spinal traction is to relax spinal musculature and to distract and separate the vertebral joint surface mechanically [40]. While the patient is in a sitting, supine, or prone position, traction is applied using electromechanical units, manual techniques, or the application of force by gravitational means. No significant difference in outcome has been demonstrated with traction vs. sham traction [41].

It is important to note, however, that spinal manipulation may be hazardous for patients with spondylosis with osteophytes impinging on nerve roots or directly on the cord. If the vertebrae are osteoporotic, traction or manipulation requires special care. Geriatric patients have a higher incidence of carotid arteriosclerosis or atherosclerosis, and sudden forceful manipulation may induce carotid artery insufficiency or the spread of emboli into the cerebral circulation.

Osteopathic manipulation therapies include the use of high-velocity, low-amplitude techniques; low-velocity, high-amplitude techniques; myofascial release; trigger point releases; and muscle energy techniques to treat somatic and visceral pain complaints. Although this therapy has proved quite effective in our practice, like most manual medicine techniques it is difficult to evaluate, in a blinded study design, the physiological effects compared to the placebo effects. As with spinal traction, osteopathic manipulation therapies should be used cautiously in the geriatric patient with suspected atherosclerotic disease, osteoporosis, and spinal stenosis.

Massage is an ancient therapy that has been growing rapidly in popularity. Classic types of massage include effleurage (stroking), petrissage (compression), tapotement (percussion), and friction. Although massage is a relatively harmless (although expensive) modality, it should be avoided in malignancy, cellulitis, lymphangitis, recent bleeding, or deep thrombosis. Specifications should also indicate whether the massage is deep or light and sedative or stimulating.

Kinematic Therapy

Kinematic therapy refers to static and dynamic body positioning. This is often quite challenging for the geriatric patient with multifactorial components of pain.

Complications of static postures and decreased movements are often sequelae of terminal illness. For numerous reasons, the patient may be unable to perform thousands of minute adjustments in posture that occur spontaneously. The patient with decreased volitional movement will need to rely on the health professional or caretaker to consistently provide these movements. Proper positioning and gentle passive range of motion can provide some measure of pain relief and decrease the complications associated with prolonged bed rest. Assisting any joint through its available range of motion activates mechanisms that reduce the intensity of pain by activating neurophysiological reflexes [24, 42]. Proper positioning can place a joint in its anatomic loose-packed position. In this position, minimal stresses are placed on the joint capsule, tendons, and muscular structures [10].

Orthotics provide a mechanism for static and dynamic positioning that allows correction of deformities, joint stabilization, decreased movement, mechanical unloading, and subsequent pain relief. Upper and lower extremity orthotics are commonly used according to the same principle as spinal orthotics. Difficulties associated with the use of orthotics in geriatric patients include difficulty donning and doffing clothing, skin breakdown, muscle atrophy, psychological dependence, nerve compression, difficulty swallowing, compliance, osteopenia, and restriction of thoracic and abdominal cavities.

Extreme care must be exercised in fitting orthotics over areas with decreased sensation or impaired circulation. These orthotics may have an impact on function by increasing energy consumption, decreasing respiratory function, and decreasing the patient's ambulation cadence or stride. These effects should be taken into account when prescribing the braces because patients with certain medical conditions (e.g., neuromuscular disease, severe deconditioning) may be unable to tolerate them.

Assistive devices provide another means of protective dynamic positioning and pain unloading. A painful or antalgic gait is characterized by avoidance of weight bearing on the involved side, shortened stance, and attempts to unload the limb as much as possible. Stability when walking and standing depends on the location of the center of gravity. Because the center of gravity plumb line or force line to the ground must fall into the area of support to make the stance stable, ground reaction pain forces may be altered by increasing the area of support. This area of support can be increased using an assistive device. An assistive device may be particularly helpful in the case of a painful lower extremity joint [43]. When using a cane to protect a painful hip joint, the cane should be held in the contralateral hand. The height of the handgrip should be positioned so that the cane can be held comfortably at an elbow flexion of 15–30°. Weight bearing should occur in a reciprocal pattern; the cane and the involved extremity bear weight simultaneously. Proper use of the cane can decrease hip joint pressure by as much as 50% [42].

Wheelchairs serve as both an assistive device and an essential orthotic for static and dynamic positioning and mobility. Unfortunately, many of the wheelchairs commonly used are designed primarily for transporting a patient from one place to another. These wheelchairs are not made for sitting in for long periods of time. The sling seats can cause the pelvis to tilt posteriorly in the sagittal plane and tilt laterally in the frontal plane creating a pelvic obliquity and spinal malalignment. The sling seat backs do not adequately support the spine which can cause excessive flexion of the lumbar spine and putting strain on muscles, ligaments, and joints [44]. Lumbar flexion also increases compressive force on the anterior vertebral bodies [44]. Excessive flexion movements have been shown to increase the risk of vertebral fractures in postmenopausal women [46]. In postmenopausal women with osteoporosis, increased spinal deformity is associated with decreased quality of life [45].

Patients with cognitive impairment or difficulty communicating may show signs of agitation or may try to get out of their wheelchair. These behaviors may, in fact, be due to pain from sitting in an uncomfortable wheelchair rather than from cognitive impairment.

Fortunately, there are many treatments that can be done to the patient and modifications to the wheelchair to improve the patient/wheelchair interface and greatly increase the patient's comfort, safety, mobility, and tolerance for sitting. Patients should be assessed and fitted with a wheelchair that fits their body and meets their sitting and mobility needs. The first step is to get the patient out of the wheelchair and onto a mat for a full physical examination to identify impairments and functional limitations and determine which problems can be addressed with treatment and which should be accommodated by modifications to the wheelchair. The wheelchair should have correct depth, width, and height and the foot pedals properly aligned. A solid seat insert with an appropriate cushion on top will provide a stable foundation for the pelvis and reduce contact pressure by distributing sitting forces over a greater area. Seat backs with additional support or curves to accommodate an excessive thoracic kyphosis can improve spinal alignment, decrease pain, improve tolerance for sitting, and help the patient to interact with the environment.

An additional kinematics modality that continues to be explored in the literature is kinesio taping. Kinesio taping is a technique based on the body's natural healing process. Whereas conventional athletic tape is designed to restrict the movement of affected muscles and joints, kinesis taping involves the use of an elastic tape designed to enhance the flow of blood and lymphatic tissues to reduce inflammation and pain. In the case of damaged muscle tissues, the tape is applied unstretched to the stretched skin of the affected areas. After application, the taped skin will form convolutions when the skin and muscles contract to their normal positions. When the skin is lifted by this technique, the flow of blood and lymphatic fluid beneath the skin improves.

The theory behind kinesis taping is that it activates neurological and circulatory systems. This method stems from the science of kinesiology; hence, the name *kinesis* is used. Muscles are not only attributed to body movements but also to circulation control of venous and lymph flows, body temperature, and so on. Therefore, the failure of the muscles to function properly induces various symptoms, including pain.

Conclusions

Despite the relative proximity of skilled nursing and rehabilitation services, the institutionalized senior continues to be at increased risk for chronic pain [47]. Although this problem has received little attention, it is anticipated that the judicious use of physical modalities and exercise, as outlined in this chapter, not only would aid in the prevention of chronic illnesses and impairment but also would decrease the need for pharmacological interventions.

The key factor of success for most physical therapy and exercise programs is enrollment and compliance. More than 50% of patients fail to complete the recommended program of exercise. Physicians can enhance the rate of compliance by establishing clear goals and objectives and by reinforcing the benefits of compliance. The most important ingredients, however, to a successful pain management program that involves active patient participation is compliance.

References

1. Lazarus BA, Murphy JB, Coletta EM, et al. The provision of physical activity to hospitalized elderly patients. Arch Intern Med. 1991;151:2452–6.
2. Kligman ED, Pepin E. Prescribing physical activity for older patients. Geriatrics. 1992;47:33–4.
3. deLateur BJ. Therapeutic exercise. In: Braddom RL, editor. Physical medicine and rehabilitation. Philadelphia: Saunders; 1996. p. 401–19.
4. Buschbacher RM. Deconditioning, conditioning, and the benefits of exercise. In: Braddom RL, editor. Physical medicine and rehabilitation. Philadelphia: Saunders; 1996. p. 687–708.
5. Hagberg JM. Effect of training on the decline of VO2max with aging. Fed Proc. 1987;46:1830–3.
6. Fiatarone MA, Marks EC, Ryan ND, et al. High-intensity strength training in nonagenarians: effects on skeletal muscle. JAMA. 1990;263:3029–34.
7. Coleman EA, Buchner DM, Cress ME, et al. The relationship of joint symptoms with exercise performance in older adults. J Am Geriatr Soc. 1996;44:14–21.
8. Ettinger WH, Burns R, Messier SP, et al. A randomized trial comparing aerobic exercise and resistance exercise with a health education program in older adults with knee osteoarthritis. JAMA. 1997;277:25–31.

9. Fisher NM, Pendergast DR, Gresham GE, et al. Muscle rehabilitation: its effects on muscular and functional performance of patients with knee osteoarthritis. Arch Phys Med Rehabil. 1991;72:367–74.

10. McCaffery M, Wolff M. Pain relief using cutaneous modalities, positioning, and movement. Hosp J. 1992;8(part 1–2):121–53.

11. Minor MA, Sanford MK. The role of physical therapy and physical modalities in pain management. Rheum Dis Clin North Am. 1999;25:233–48.

12. Koh TC. Tai chi chuan. Am J Chin Med. 1981;9(11):15–22.

13. Koh TC. Tai chi and ankylosing spondylitis – a personal experience. Am J Chin Med. 1982;10(1–4):59–61.

14. Kirsteins AE, Dietz F, Hwang SM. Evaluating the safety and potential use of a weight-bearing exercise, tai-chi chuan, for rheumatoid arthritis patients. Am J Phys Med Rehabil. 1991;70(3):136–41.

15. Ozgönenel L, Aytekin E, Durmu oglu G. A double-blind trial of clinical effects of therapeutic ultrasound in knee osteoarthritis. Ultrasound Med Biol. 2009;35(1):44–9.

16. Srbely JZ, Dickey JP, Lowerison M, Edwards AM, Nolet PS, Wong LL. Stimulation of myofascial trigger points with ultrasound induces segmental antinociceptive effects: a randomized controlled study. Pain. 2008;139(2):260–6.

17. Srbely JZ, Dickey JP. Randomized controlled study of the antinociceptive effect of ultrasound on trigger point sensitivity: novel applications in myofascial therapy? Clin Rehabil. 2007;21(5):411–7.

18. Srbely JZ. Ultrasound in the management of osteoarthritis: part I: a review of the current literature. J Can Chiropr Assoc. 2008;52(1):30–7.

19. Thamsborg G, Florescu A, Oturai P, Fallentin E, Tritsaris K, Dissing S. Treatment of knee osteoarthritis with pulsed electromagnetic fields: a randomized, double-blind, placebo-controlled study. Osteoarthritis Cartilage. 2005;13(7):575–81.

20. Cetin N, Aytar A, Atalay A, Akman MN. Comparing hot pack, short-wave diathermy, ultrasound, and TENS on isokinetic strength, pain, and functional status of women with osteoarthritic knees: a single-blind, randomized, controlled trial. Am J Phys Med Rehabil. 2008;87(6):443–51.

21. Dogru H, Basaran S, Sarpel T. Effectiveness of therapeutic ultrasound in adhesive capsulitis. Joint Bone Spine. 2008;75(4):445–50.

22. Warden SJ, Metcalf BR, Kiss ZS, Cook JL, Purdam CR, Bennell KL, et al. Low-intensity pulsed ultrasound for chronic patellar tendinopathy: a randomized, double-blind, placebo-controlled trial. Rheumatology (Oxford). 2008;47(4):467–71.

23. Rattanachaiyanont M, Kuptniratsaikul V. No additional benefit of shortwave diathermy over exercise program for knee osteoarthritis in peri-/post-menopausal women: an equivalence trial. Osteoarthritis Cartilage. 2008;16(7):823–8.

24. Clark GR, Willis LA, Stenner L, et al. Evaluation of physiotherapy in the treatment of osteoarthritis of the knee. Rheumatol Rehabil. 1974;13:190–7.

25. Hecht PJ, Bachmann S, Booth RE, et al. Effects of thermal therapy on rehabilitation after total knee arthroplasty. A prospective randomized study. Clin Orthop. 1983;178:198–201.

26. Angilaski J. Baggie therapy: simple relief for arthritic knees. JAMA. 1981;24:317.

27. Williams, Harvey J, Tannenbaum H. Use of superficial heat versus ice for the rheumatoid arthritic shoulder. A pilot study. Physiother Can. 1986;38:6.

28. Schwab CB, editor. Musculoskeletal pain. Phys Med Rehabil. 1991;5(3):1.

29. Michlovitz SL. Biophysical principles of hearing and superficial heat agents. In: Michlovitz SL, editor. Thermal agents in rehabilitation. Philadelphia: Davis. 1987;107–111.

30. Draper D, Prentice W. In: Prentice WE, editor. Therapeutic modalities for physical therapists, 2nd ed. New York: McGraw-Hill; 2002. Chap. 10, p. 263–306.

31. Deyo RA, Walsh NE, Martin DC, et al. A controlled trial of transcutaneous electrical nerve stimulation (TENS) and exercise for chronic low back pain. N Engl J Med. 1990;322: 1627–34.

32. Garland D, Holt P, Harrington JT, Caldwell J, Zizic T, Cholewczynski J. A 3-month, randomized, double-blind, placebo-controlled study to evaluate the safety and efficacy of a highly optimized,

capacitively coupled, pulsed electrical stimulator in patients with osteoarthritis of the knee. Osteoarthritis Cartilage. 2007;15(6):630–7.

33. Zizic TM, Hoffman KC, Holt PA, Hungerford DS, O'Dell JR, Jacobs MA, et al. The treatment of osteoarthritis of the knee with pulsed electrical stimulation. J Rheumatol. 1995;22(9):1757–61.

34. Mont MA, Hungerford DS, Caldwell JR, Ragland PS, Hoffman KC, He YD, Jones LC, Zizic TM. Pulsed electrical stimulation to defer TKA in patients with knee osteoarthritis. Orthopedics. 2006;29(10):887–92.

35. Bjordal JM, Johnson MI, Lopes-Martins RA, Bogen B, Chow R, Ljunggren AE. Short-term efficacy of physical interventions in osteoarthritic knee pain. A systematic review and meta-analysis of randomised placebo-controlled trials. BMC Musculoskelet Disord. 2007;8:51.

36. Poitras S, Brosseau L. Evidence-informed management of chronic low back pain with transcutaneous electrical nerve stimulation, interferential current, electrical muscle stimulation, ultrasound, and thermotherapy. Spine J. 2008;8(1):226–33. Review.

37. Zambito A, Bianchini D, Gatti D, Rossini M, Adami S, Viapiana O. Interferential and horizontal therapies in chronic low back pain due to multiple vertebral fractures: a randomized, double blind, clinical study. Osteoporos Int. 2007;18(11):1541–5.

38. Zambito A, Bianchini D, Gatti D, Viapiana O, Rossini M, Adami S. Interferential and horizontal therapies in chronic low back pain: a randomized,double blind, clinical study. Clin Exp Rheumatol. 2006;24(5):534–9.

39. Semalty A, Semalty M, Singh R, Saraf SK, Saraf S. Iontophoretic drug delivery system: a review. Technol Health Care. 2007;15(4):237–45.

40. Bengston R. Physical measures useful in pain management. Int Anesthesiol Clin. 1983;21:165–76.

41. Malanga GA, Nadler SF. Nonoperative treatment of low back pain. Mayo Clin Proc. 1999;74:1135–48.

42. Neumann DA. Biomechanical analysis of selected principles of hip joint protection. Arthritis Care Res. 1989;2:146–55.

43. Lehman JF, Lehman JF, editors. Krusen's handbook of physical medicine and rehabilitation. Philadelphia: Saunders; 1990. p. 108–125.

44. Pynt J, Mackey MG, Higgs J. Kyphosed seated postures: extending concepts of postural health beyond the office. J Occup Rehabil. 2008;18(1):35–45.

45. Miyakoshi N, Itoi E, Kobayashi M, Kodama H. Impact of postural deformities and spinal mobility on quality of life in postmenopausal osteoporosis. Osteoporos Int. 2003; 14:1007–12.

46. Sinaki M, Mikkelsen BA. Postmenopausal spinal osteoporosis: flexion versus extension exercises. Arch Phys Med Rehabil. 1984;65(10):593–6.

47. Sengstaken EA, King SA. The problems of pain and its detection among geriatric nursing home residents. J Am Geriatr Soc. 1993;41:541.

Chapter 7
Pharmacotherapy of Pain in Older Adults: Nonopioid

Mary Lynn McPherson and Tanya J. Uritsky

> *The desire to take medicine is one feature which distinguishes man, the animal from his fellow creatures.*
>
> Sir William Osler

With approximately 80% of visits to physicians involving conditions with a painful component and at least 50 million Americans suffering from chronic pain, it is imperative to have an appreciation of pharmacotherapies available for treating pain [1, 2]. Pain medications account for the second most prescribed class of drugs (after cardiac-renal drugs), making up 12% of all medications prescribed during ambulatory office visits in the USA [3]. The National Institutes of Health have estimated chronic pain to be the third largest health problem in the world [4]. Chronic pain is a problem that will become increasingly more prevalent as the US population aged 65 and older rapidly increases, as it is predicted to exceed 70 million by the year 2030 [2]. As many as 80% of older persons with cancer experience pain during the course of their illness [5]. The first chapter of this book makes it clear that complaints of pain are particularly common among older adults, occurring twice as often in persons over 65 years of age as compared to younger people [6–8].

Despite growing understanding of the pathogenesis of pain and the availability of a wide variety of treatment options, older adults are not receiving adequate pain relief. Pitkala et al. determined that only one-third of home-dwelling older adults suffering from daily pain that interfered with functioning had been prescribed any type of regular analgesic drug in 1999 [9]. Overall, only one-quarter of patients with daily pain received analgesics of any kind. Of the patients who were prescribed an analgesic, 25% received a World Health Organization (WHO) level 1 drug (nonopioid); 6% a WHO level 2 drug (weak opioid), and 3% a WHO level 3 drug (strong opioid). Patients over 85 years of age, nonwhite patients, and patients with cognitive impairment were at greater risk for receiving no analgesics [10].

M.L. McPherson (✉)
Department of Pharmacy Practice and Science, University of Maryland School of Pharmacy, 20 N. Pine Street, Room 405, Baltimore, Maryland 21201, USA
e-mail: mmcphers@rx.umaryland.edu

F.M. Gloth, III (ed.), *Handbook of Pain Relief in Older Adults: An Evidence-Based Approach*, Aging Medicine, DOI 10.1007/978-1-60761-618-4_7,
© Springer Science+Business Media, LLC 2011

Cognitive impairment likely contributes to the undertreatment of pain due to the inherent difficulties in recognizing and assessing pain in these patients.

Inadequate pain management is a problem in nursing facilities as well. In a 3-month retrospective drug utilization evaluation performed by consultant pharmacists on selected analgesics used in nursing facilities, it was found that there was a lack of adequate pain assessment and inappropriate use of analgesic medications [11]. Of the 2,542 patients receiving opioids or nonsteroidal anti-inflammatory drugs (NSAIDs), 67.6% were for opioids, 24.8% were for NSAIDs, and 7.6% were for tramadol [11]. Propoxyphene-containing drugs were considered as part of the opioid group and were the most frequently prescribed of all analgesics (35.6%). Most analgesics, 63.2%, were prescribed on an as needed basis [11]. These practices are inconsistent with recommended pain therapy in older people.

Underreported and undertreated pain may result in serious consequences to psychological and physical functioning and overall quality of life in older adults. The goal of pain management in older adults is to reduce or eliminate the complaint of pain to a mutually accepted level that allows the patient to improve overall functional status and minimize adverse effects from analgesics. Although most older adults require analgesics to treat pain, nonpharmacologic interventions, such as those described in the previous chapter, should be utilized whenever possible. The evidence is particularly strong for patient and caregiver education, cognitive-behavioral therapy, application of heat or cold, osteopathic manipulative treatment, exercise programs, and counseling [12]. Additionally, a thorough interdisciplinary assessment may help to identify contributing factors, such as cultural and psychological reasons for the pain. When nonpharmacologic interventions are insufficient to control pain alone, pharmacologic therapy should be instituted, after carefully assessing the patient, and individualizing therapy. "Rational polypharmacy," or the prescribing of more than a single agent, may be necessary and may even work synergistically to provide greater relief with less toxicity than would higher doses of a single agent [5].

Factors to Consider

General Considerations

Pharmacotherapy in older adults is complicated by a narrower therapeutic index (dosage range between therapeutic efficacy and toxicity) for most medications, as compared to that in younger individuals. Epidemiological studies of adverse drug reactions (ADRs) have attempted to determine whether age alone increases the risk for adverse drug outcomes. While controversial, the trend seems to be that advancing age does increase the risk of experiencing an adverse drug effect [13]. Beyth and Shorr propose, however, that the probability of a patient developing an ADR is multifactorial, reflecting the agent (the drug, dose, and duration of therapy), the host (age, measures of severity of illness, nursing home residence, or recent hospital discharge), and the environment (generalist vs. specialist prescriber) [13]. Additional risk factors for ADRs have been identified as inappropriate medication selection and the use of multiple medications (polypharmacy) [14]. A recent study by Jonell and Klarin revealed a strong association between the number of dispensed drugs and the probability of a clinically relevant (26%) or potentially serious (5%) drug–drug interaction in people aged 75 years and older [14].

Perception of Pain in the Older Adult

With advancing age, the perception of pain is altered. It is thought that this is due, at least in part, to brain atrophy as well as some other mechanisms that contribute to a lower pain threshold [2]. The older person's experience of pain may be altered because of impaired descending inhibition of the pain signal. It has been shown in younger patients that fear, dysfunctional coping, depression, and anxiety lead to impaired descending inhibition which contributes to disability in persistent pain conditions [15]. Accordingly, these age-related changes contribute to a diminished ability of the patient to effectively respond to the stress of persistent pain. Additional contributing factors include decreased cognitive reserves, decreased density of opioid receptors, polypharmacy, high medical comorbidities, frequent social isolation, and depression [15].

Pharmacokinetic Considerations

Physiologic changes associated with aging may alter the way the body handles a medication, including opioids and other analgesics. These changes contribute to narrowing the therapeutic range of analgesics, and increase the risk for drug-induced toxicity.

Absorption: Drug absorption is probably the least affected by aging of all the pharmacokinetic processes. Older adults produce less saliva, which may be further reduced by the administration of medications with anticholinergic properties [17]. The result is a delay in the absorption of sublingual tablets and matrix-embedded formulations [17]. Older adults may also experience increased gastric pH, decreased gastric surface area, decreased intestinal blood flow, and reduced gastrointestinal motility [13]. These changes associated with aging generally do not significantly influence analgesic therapy; however, slowed motility may increase gastrointestinal irritation, bleeding, and ulceration secondary to NSAID agents [16].

Distribution: Aging is usually associated with a decrease in total body water and lean body mass and an increase in total body fat. This shift in the lean:fat body mass ratio affects the distribution of drugs throughout the body by decreasing the volume of distribution for a hydrophilic drug (i.e., morphine) and increasing the volume of distribution of a lipophilic drug (i.e., fentanyl) [13]. This results in high serum peaks (which may cause toxicity) and slower decrease in plasma concentration (longer duration of action) of water-soluble drugs and an increased risk of accumulation and slightly delayed onset of action with lipid-soluble drugs [16].

Many drugs, including analgesics, are extensively bound to plasma proteins, such as albumin. Older adults may produce less albumin, particularly in the presence of concurrent disease, immobility, or poor nutrition [13]. The consequence of reduced plasma proteins is a higher "unbound" or "free fraction" of drug, which is then available to effect the pharmacologic, and by extension, the toxic effect of the medication. Therapy with opioids, NSAIDs, benzodiazepines, and phenytoin may result in a heightened therapeutic response, or toxicity in patients with hypoalbuminemia [16].

Metabolism: Many medications, including analgesics, are detoxified by the liver. In older adults, functional liver tissue diminishes and hepatic blood flow decreases. Hepatic enzyme activity may be diminished in the cytochrome P450 system. Subsequently, hepatic metabolism is reduced by 30–40% [17]. Reduced hepatic extraction results in increased oral bioavailability of some opioids [17]. The clinical implication of these effects is possible accumulation of the parent drug (e.g., NSAID, opioid, and benzodiazepine), anticipating the need for lower dosing, and/or prolonged dosing intervals [13, 16].

Elimination: While there is considerable interindividual variability, renal function generally declines with aging. Every year over the age of 50, renal function decreases by 1% [17]. The decline includes a reduction in renal mass and blood flow, and a decline in glomerular filtration and tubular reabsorption rates [16]. The majority of drugs and/or their metabolites are eliminated from the body by the kidneys. Older adults are at risk for drug accumulation when the drug has a long half-life, the parent drug is renally eliminated, or the renally eliminated drug metabolites are pharmacologically active. Even within one group of analgesics, there may be preferred agents for patients with renal impairment. For example, morphine is metabolized to pharmacologically active drug products that are renally eliminated and may result in toxicity with accumulation. Should this occur, a better choice of opioid may be hydromorphone or oxycodone, opioids whose metabolites have negligible activity [13].

Other Considerations: A decrease in sympathetic innervation of the juxtaglomerular cells within the kidney in the older adult results in decreased production of renin and aldosterone. This puts older adults at an increased risk for hyperkalemia, especially with NSAIDS, in the face of decreased renin production. There is also an age-related diminished baroreceptor response that puts the older adult at increased risk for orthostasis with medications such as tricyclic antidepressants and phenothiazines [17].

Pharmacodynamic Considerations

Pharmacodynamics refers to the effect of the medication on the body, both the pharmacologic response and the magnitude of the response. While there is significant interpatient variability of the pharmacokinetics and pharmacodynamics of opioid therapy, it does seem that older adults are more sensitive to the effects of analgesics, particularly opioids [18]. Single-dose studies of opioids used for postoperative and cancer pain have shown greater pain relief and a longer duration of action in older adults than in younger adults [14, 19]. Despite the controversy of whether this effect is due to altered pharmacodynamics, or due to pharmacokinetic changes, it would be prudent to heed the advice, "start low and go slow" when dosing analgesics in older adults.

Comorbid States

Diseases that are commonly experienced by older adults may further adversely affect changes in the pharmacokinetics or pharmacodynamics of analgesics. Diseases that adversely affect renal or hepatic function may further complicate the metabolism and/or excretion of analgesics. For example, chronic liver disease and congestive heart failure may reduce hepatic blood flow, resulting in diminished hepatic metabolism of some analgesics, drug accumulation, and possible toxicity. Older adults with preexisting dementia may be at increased risk for increased somnolence and cognitive impairment with opioid therapy [13]. Comorbid depression worsens disability and decreases active coping in patients suffering from pain. It also decreases the likelihood that either condition will respond favorably to treatment and diminishes patient satisfaction with the drug therapy [3]. The comorbidity of anxiety with pain appears to be nearly as significant as that of comorbid depression. A study of 85,000 community-dwelling adults conducted by the WHO in 2008 found that the prevalence of mood and anxiety disorders was positively correlated with increasing number of pain sites [3].

Patients with multiple chronic diseases are likely to take multiple medications. Polypharmacy increases the likelihood that a patient will experience a drug-related problem [20]. Medications that adversely affect the central nervous system may result in an exaggerated effect when taken with opioids. Similarly, taking an NSAID with other gastrotoxic agents increases the risk for toxicity.

Other Considerations

Older adults frequently are nonadherent to prescribed drug therapy for a variety of reasons. This behavior may be unintentional secondary to a complex medication regimen, misunderstanding of prescribing instructions, or cognitive deficits or physical impairments such as vision or hearing loss [15]. On the other hand, nonadherence may be purposeful in response to lack of interest, experiencing adverse effects from analgesics, fears about continued use of opioids, or inability to pay for the medications. It is imperative that practitioners streamline the analgesic regimen to enhance adherence; nonadherence to drug therapy is the ultimate absorption barrier. Issues of secondary gain, focusing on the complaint of pain, prior experience with pain and analgesic therapy, and concurrent anxiety should be explored, and evaluated in terms of impacting pain treatment [21].

Nonopioid Therapy

Acetaminophen

Mechanism of Action

Acetaminophen acts by inhibiting prostaglandin synthesis in the central nervous system, resulting in an analgesic and antipyretic effect similar to that seen with aspirin therapy. Unlike aspirin, however, acetaminophen is a weak prostaglandin inhibitor in the periphery, and possesses no significant anti-inflammatory properties [22]. It cannot be said that acetaminophen lacks anti-inflammatory effects completely, as it has been shown to effectively reduce the inflammation following oral surgery, similar to that of the NSAID ibuprofen [23].

There was some early evidence that acetaminophen may act by inhibiting a variant of the enzyme cyclooxygenase, which researchers have labeled cyclooxygenase-3 or "COX-3" [24, 25]. When COX-3 was isolated in canines in 2002, it appeared that acetaminophen may target the cells with COX-3 in those animals, and so it was theorized that this was the case in humans as well [25]. Additional research has demonstrated that the COX-3 enzyme is an unlikely target of acetaminophen and recent DNA studies have found that it is very unlikely that active COX-3 could exist in human tissues [25]. The cyclooxygenase enzyme seems to be involved in the synthesis of prostaglandins, which play many roles throughout the body, including mediation of pain and inflammation. As will be discussed in the NSAID section of this chapter, researchers have discovered that there are at least two variations of the COX enzyme: 1 and 2. It is thought that acetaminophen is a selective inhibitor of the COX-2 enzyme, demonstrating similar pharmacological effects of analgesia and antipyresis and lack of gastrointestinal aggravation associated with COX-1 inhibition [23]. When levels of arachadonic acid are low, COX-2 is responsible for the production of low-level prostaglandin activity in cells. Acetaminophen is thought to target these low-turnover cells [23]. There is increasing evidence as well that analgesic properties may be due in part to the inhibition of the prostaglandin synthesis in combination with supraspinal activation of descending serotonergic pathways [23].

Place in Therapy

Acetaminophen may be administered as monotherapy for the treatment of mild pain, or in combination with other nonopioids such as aspirin, caffeine, salicylamide, and others. Results of studies evaluating pain relief from these acetaminophen/

nonopioid combination products have been conflicting. Acetaminophen combined with aspirin and caffeine may be more effective than acetaminophen alone in the treatment of tension headaches, but acetaminophen combined with aspirin, caffeine, or salicylamide generally has not been shown to be more effective than optimized dosages of acetaminophen alone, nor has combination therapy been shown to cause fewer adverse effects [26]. Acetaminophen (650 mg doses) in combination with an opioid (i.e., hydrocodone, codeine, or oxycodone) may be used to treat moderate pain, as the therapeutic effect shown from combination therapy exceeds that of either analgesic alone or that achieved by increasing the opioid dose [26].

Acetaminophen is usually the first drug of choice for the treatment of mild-to-moderate pain in older adults due to its low cost, therapeutic efficacy, and safety profile. The American Medical Directors Association (AMDA) Clinical Practice Guidelines for "Chronic Pain Management in the Long-Term Care Setting" recommend the use of acetaminophen as a first-line analgesic for mild-to-moderate pain in older adults, if they do not have liver disease or consume excess amounts of alcohol [27]. The American Geriatrics Society (AGS) provided updated guidelines for "The Management of Persistent Pain in Older Persons" in 2009, advocating for acetaminophen in as an initial and ongoing therapy in the treatment of persistent, and more specifically musculoskeletal, pain with dosage reduction in patients with organ dysfunction or hazardous or harmful alcohol use [5].

Osteoarthritis is a painful disorder that is highly prevalent in older adults. Amadio and Cummings evaluated acetaminophen 4,000 mg/day vs. placebo in 25 patients with osteoarthritis of the knee [28]. Acetaminophen resulted in significant improvements in both pain at rest and on motion, and on physician and patient global assessment. Bradley et al. demonstrated equivalent pain relief with acetaminophen 4,000 mg/day and ibuprofen 2,400 mg/day; however, joint inflammation was more responsive to ibuprofen than to acetaminophen [29]. Williams et al. compared acetaminophen 2,600 mg/day and naproxen 750 mg/day in 178 patients with osteoarthritis of the knee [30]. The authors concluded that the two regimens had similar efficacy, although it was slightly better for naproxen.

A Cochrane review of NSAID vs. acetaminophen therapy for osteoarthritis found that NSAIDs were associated with improved pain and function but that acetaminophen appears to be as safe as placebo and safer than traditional NSAIDs in terms of GI effects [31]. Benefits of NSAIDs over acetaminophen are mostly associated with moderate-to-severe baseline pain levels [31]. Another meta-analysis done comparing the efficacy and safety of NSAID agents vs. acetaminophen in the treatment of osteoarthritis of the hip or knee found similar results. It concluded that NSAIDs, including COX-2 inhibitors, are superior to acetaminophen in reducing rest and walking pain in patients with symptomatic osteoarthritis, although this increased analgesic efficacy was modest and accompanied by a trend for a higher level of withdrawals due to adverse effects in the NSAID-treatment group [32]. Safety results must be interpreted with caution as randomized controlled trials have been relatively short in duration and studied a small number of highly selected participants with osteoarthritis, and so results are not likely generalizable to a more heterogeneous population [31]. Given the modest benefits of NSAIDs over acetaminophen, it is imperative to consider patient preference, clinical judgments, cost, accessibility, and safety risks of both agents in the individual patient [31].

The American College of Rheumatology recommends acetaminophen for mild-to-moderate osteoarthritis joint pain as an initial intervention [33]. The 2002 guidelines of The American Pain Society also recommend acetaminophen as the analgesic of first choice for mild osteoarthritis pain, and continued therapy for patients who experience a favorable risk-to-benefit ratio [34]. Newer guidelines from the Osteoarthritis Research Society International (OARSI) recommend acetaminophen, up to 4 g/day, as initial therapy for mild-to-moderate pain in patients with hip or knee osteoarthritis [35].

Adverse Effects/Precautions

Acetaminophen is usually well tolerated and has no common adverse effects when used in therapeutic doses of no more than 4,000 mg/day [36]. Patients receiving acetaminophen in the trials described above experienced no serious drug-related adverse effects [37]. Bannwarth et al. evaluated both single and multiple dose pharmacokinetics of acetaminophen in polymedicated very old patients with rheumatic pain [38]. Patients were 89 years old on average, and taking 3–8 concomitant medications. Pharmacokinetic parameters were derived from a single dose of 1,000 mg acetaminophen, and after receiving 1,000 mg three times daily for 5 consecutive days. The investigators observed no drug accumulation with multiple doses of acetaminophen as compared to single doses and concluded that 1,000 mg three times daily is safe for older adults.

Some studies have suggested that chronic ingestion of acetaminophen increases the risk of chronic renal disease [39]. Perneger et al. concluded that patients taking an average of more than one acetaminophen tablet per day, or a cumulative acetaminophen intake of more than 1,000 tablets per lifetime doubled the odds of developing end-stage renal disease [40]. Despite these data, the Scientific Advisory Committee of the National Kidney Foundation recommends that acetaminophen be used as the analgesic of choice in patients with impaired renal function [41, 42].

Hepatic toxicity rarely occurs with daily acetaminophen doses of 4,000 mg/day or less, however higher daily doses taken chronically, or concurrent ethanol consumption increases the risk of acetaminophen-induced hepatotoxicity [1, 43, 44]. It appears that the transient elevations of alanine aminotransferase that have been observed in long-term patients do not directly translate into liver failure or hepatic dysfunction when maximum recommended doses are avoided [5]. Regardless, in September 2002, the FDA's Nonprescription Drugs Advisory Committee suggested that acetaminophen labeling should be changed to include a liver damage warning separate from the current "alcohol warning" [45]. Although warnings about the toxicity of acetaminophen have been strengthened, intentional and unintentional overdoses continue to occur, most likely as a result of consumer unawareness or lack of concern [14]. Cham et al. surveyed 213 subjects who presented in the Emergency Department on their basic knowledge about nonprescription analgesics [46].

Sixty-four percent of respondents did not know acetaminophen use may result in liver toxicity. One study conducted between 1995 and 2004 found that the incidence of overdose cases in the elderly was 4.5% [14]. Patients and prescribers alike need to be mindful of the ubiquitous nature of acetaminophen in multiple-ingredient prescription and nonprescription medications. For example, Vicodin ES (extra strength) caplets contain 7.5 mg hydrocodone and 750 mg acetaminophen. If a patient consumed two caplets every 4 h around the clock, this would result in a total daily acetaminophen dose of 9,000 mg. Similarly, many multisymptom relieving nonprescription products contain acetaminophen.

At the time of writing, appropriate use of acetaminophen in older adults with normal renal and hepatic function, and no history of alcohol abuse is a maximum total daily dose of 4,000 mg/day. The AGS guidelines recommend reduction of the maximum acetaminophen dosage by 50–75%, or selection of alternate therapy in patients with hepatic insufficiency or a history of alcohol abuse [5]. The Guidelines for the Acute Pain Management in Older Adults (2006) from the University of Iowa recommend doses of no more than 4 g/day in general with a reduction to a maximum of 3 g/day in frail elderly [47]. Lastly, the AMDA guidelines recommend a maximum dosage of 3,000 mg every 24 h for elderly patients in the long-term care setting, with a consideration of a daily maximum of 2,000 mg for patients with renal or hepatic impairment [27].

Recently, in 2008, the FDA Acetaminophen Hepatotoxicity Working Group recommended limiting the maximum individual acetaminophen dosage unit to 325 mg instead of 500 mg, with a maximum single adult dose of 650 mg of acetaminophen instead of a single 1,000 mg dose [48]. They also recommended decreasing the maximum total daily dose to 3,250 mg instead of 4,000 mg/day [48]. A joint meeting in June 2009 of the Drug and Safety Risk Management, Anesthetic and Life Support Drugs and the Nonprescription Drugs advisory committees of the FDA recommended banning combination opioid and acetaminophen products, increasing warnings regarding potential liver damage, reducing individual doses to 325 mg and an overall decrease of the total daily dose to less than 4,000 mg, although a specific daily maximum was not recommended [48]. They also recommended requiring a prescription for dosage units of more than 325 mg and limiting the number of pills per container [48].

Although acetaminophen does not affect platelet function, it may cause elevation of the prothrombin time in warfarin-treated patients, especially with higher doses of each drug [48].

Doses greater than 2 g/day for at least 1 week are associated with elevations in the international normalized ratio [48]. Patients should be advised to limit therapy to short-term treatment of acute illnesses in light of this interaction.

Summary

In summary, acetaminophen is an effective analgesic for mild-to-moderate pain in older adults. While acetaminophen will treat the pain associated with inflammatory disease states, it will not noticeably reduce inflammation. Close attention should be paid to acetaminophen dosing, not exceeding the currently recommended 4,000 mg/day, and giving consideration to a limit of 3,000 mg/day in the frail elderly. Patients at risk for acetaminophen toxicity, such as those who use alcohol or have liver disease, should not receive acetaminophen. The FDA is considering regulation of combination products for both controlled prescription medications and OTC preparations regarding safety for public use.

Nonsteroidal Anti-inflammatory Drugs

Mechanism of Action

NSAIDs are one of the most widely prescribed groups of medications worldwide. In 2000, 70% of adults over age 65 were taking NSAIDs at least once a week [50, 51]. NSAIDs exhibit antipyretic and analgesic activity as seen with acetaminophen, but also exhibit more potent anti-inflammatory properties. Many painful conditions that affect older adults have an inflammatory component, particularly arthritis (rheumatoid more so than osteoarthritis). The NSAIDs also reduce swelling, tenderness, and stiffness, allowing for improved overall physical functioning [52]. Up to 25% of ambulatory older adults use prescription strength NSAIDs each year; an even greater percentage of older adults may actually be using NSAIDs regularly, if nonprescription strength NSAIDs are also considered [53].

NSAIDs act by inhibiting the synthesis of prostaglandins. Arachidonic acid is the primary precursor of prostaglandins and is metabolized by either the lipoxygenase pathway to leukotrienes or via the cyclooxygenase pathway to prostaglandins, thromboxanes, and prostacyclins. Two cylcooxygenase isoforms have been identified: cyclooxygenase-1 (COX-1) and cyclooxygenase-2 (COX-2). COX-1 is found in most normal cells and tissues and is considered to be homeostatic in function, while COX-2 is induced in inflammatory settings by cytokines and inflammatory mediators. COX-2 is also constitutively expressed in certain areas of the kidney and brain. COX-1 leads to the production of prostaglandins and thromboxanes responsible for gastrointestinal mucosal integrity, platelet aggregation, and renal function. COX-2 leads to the production of prostaglandins responsible for inflammation as well as other functions such as mitogenesis and growth, regulation of female reproduction, bone formation, and renal function [54, 55].

Older NSAIDs such as aspirin, ibuprofen, naproxen, and others are nonselective inhibitors of the two isoforms of the cyclooxygenase enzyme (e.g., they inhibit both COX-1 and COX-2 isoenzymes). Unsurprisingly, the adverse effects associated with nonselective NSAID therapy are an extension of the pharmacologic effect, and include dyspepsia, epigastric distress, nausea, erosion or ulceration of the GI mucosa, inhibition of platelet aggregation and prolonged bleeding time, deterioration of renal function, overt renal decompensation, and acute tubular necrosis with renal failure [56].

NSAIDs with greater selectivity for COX-2 than COX-1 have been developed to treat pain and inflammation with fewer gastrointestinal adverse effects than nonselective NSAIDs. At this time, celecoxib is the only COX-2 selective NSAID available: rofecoxib and valdecoxib were removed from the market in 2004 and 2005, respectively. These agents have the analgesic, anti-inflammatory, and antipyretic activities of nonspecific NSAIDs, but are less toxic to the gastrointestinal system. There is evidence demonstrating that selective COX-2 inhibitors are associated with significantly less gastrointestinal adverse effects, but may have more risk for cardiovascular events. Inhibition of COX-2 is thought to shift the balance in enzyme activity to COX-1, resulting in an increase in thromboxane A2 (prothrombotic) relative to prostacyclin (vasodilator and platelet inhibitor) and subsequent platelet aggregation, vasoconstriction and prothrombotic events [14].

Increased cardiovascular risk is associated with both COX-2 selective and nonselective NSAID agents. McGettigan and Henry performed a systematic review of observational studies of COX-2 and nonselective NSAIDs [57]. The analysis revealed that celecoxib, in doses of 200 mg/day, was not associated with an increased cardiovascular risk [relative risk (RR) 1.06], an effect that seems to be lost at higher doses (400 mg daily or greater). Diclofenac and indomethacin, at commonly used doses, were both associated with an increased risk of cardiovascular events, RR 1.36 and 1.40, respectively, equivalent to that seen with rofecoxib. Ibuprofen and naproxen did not seem to be associated with an increased risk of cardiovascular events (RR 1.09 and 0.99, respectively) [57].

Place in Therapy

NSAIDs play a major role in the management of acute and chronic pain experienced by older adults, especially syndromes with an inflammatory component. NSAIDs reduce joint pain and stiffness with both osteoarthritis and rheumatoid arthritis, and tenderness and swelling associated with rheumatoid arthritis. NSAIDs are also effective at reducing pain in acute gout, bursitis, tendonitis, seronegative spondyloarthropathies, soft tissue injuries, and postsurgical pain [53]. All NSAID and COX-2 agents appear equally effective in the treatment of pain disorders [3, 50].

The Agency for Health Care Policy and Research (AHCPR) guidelines for "Acute Pain Management: Operative or Medical Procedures and Trauma" published in 1992 recommend that the pharmacologic management of mild-to-moderate postoperative pain should begin with NSAID therapy, unless there is a contraindication [58]. Further, the guidelines advocate for the use of NSAIDs alone after relatively noninvasive surgery. If NSAID therapy alone is insufficient, it is reasonable to administer the NSAID along with an opioid, resulting in an "opioid-sparing" effect, and reducing opioid side effects. The concurrent use of opioids and NSAIDs often provides more effective analgesia than either of the drug classes alone [58]. NSAIDs have been shown to be useful in treating acute pain from gall bladder and urinary tract spasms where opioids may have relatively less effect [59].

Ketorolac (Toradol) is a nonselective NSAID and is the only NSAID available in the USA for parenteral administration. This agent is useful in acute pain situations such as trauma or surgery when oral analgesic therapy is not feasible. Ketorolac has even been used preoperatively as a preemptive analgesic with good results [60]. Ketorolac may be used safely in older adults unable to take oral nonopioids when certain considerations are addressed. Ketorolac is contraindicated in frail older adults with dehydration, preexisting renal dysfunction, cirrhosis, or heart failure. The dose should be decreased by 50% of the recommended dose for younger individuals, should not exceed 60 mg daily, and should not be used for longer than 5 days at a time [47].

Several studies have compared the analgesic efficacy of the nonselective NSAIDs vs. celecoxib in the management of acute pain. Celecoxib is approved for the management of acute pain in the USA. A recent study evaluated the analgesic efficacy of celecoxib 400 mg vs. ibuprofen 400 mg in the treatment of acute dental pain [61]. Although there was no difference in the onset of analgesia or level of analgesia achieved, patients who received celecoxib maintained analgesia for a significantly longer period of time [61]. A Cochrane Review of eight trials of single dose oral celecoxib in the treatment of acute postoperative pain in adults found similar results. Celecoxib 400 mg was found to be at least as effective as ibuprofen 400 mg and provided a longer duration of pain relief than both ibuprofen and diclofenac, but not naproxen [62].

NSAID agents have been shown to be effective in the treatment of mild-to-moderate chronic pain, particularly those conditions associated with inflammation. The majority of prescriptions written for NSAID therapy in older adults are for the treatment of pain and/or inflammation due to arthritis. Historically osteoarthritis (OA) was not considered an inflammatory process until the disease reached an advanced stage; however, others have suggested that OA may be associated with local low-grade inflammation [63–65].

Recently, Singh et al. performed a study comparing celecoxib with naproxen and diclofenac in patients with osteoarthritis [66]. Patients were assigned to celecoxib 100 or 200 mg twice daily, diclofenac 50 mg twice daily, or naproxen 500 mg twice daily for 12 weeks. Celecoxib was proven to be equally effective in the treatment of OA as the nonselective agents but was associated with significantly fewer serious upper gastrointestinal events and no significant difference in the number of cardiovascular events [66].

Topical NSAID agents also provide effective peripheral anti-inflammatory benefits with a 17 times lower systemic exposure compared with oral administration and 158 times lower average peak plasma concentration [67]. Diclofenac sodium gel is approved for the treatment of osteoarthritis (OA) pain. Diclofenac gel demonstrated significant improvement for pain over placebo in the treatment of OA of the knee at up to 12 weeks of treatment [67]. Although there is the risk of side effects associated with systemic NSAIDs, trials have shown that most frequent side effects include reactions at the application site [67]. There was no report of GI side effects [67]. The OARSI guidelines recommend topical NSAID agents as possible effective alternatives and adjunct agents in OA of the knee [35].

The AGS guidelines for the treatment of persistent pain in older adults recommend that nonselective NSAID and COX-2 selective inhibitors be considered rarely and with extreme caution in highly selected patients [5]. Patient selection should include those who have failed safer alternative therapies, continually fail to meet therapeutic goals and in whom ongoing assessment of therapeutic benefit outweighs risk of complications. Absolute contraindications for NSAID use are active peptic ulcer disease, chronic kidney disease, and heart failure [5]. Relative contraindications include hypertension, *Heliobacter pylori*, history of peptic ulcer disease, and concomitant use of corticosteroids or selective serotonin reuptake inhibitors [5]. Older persons taking a nonselective NSAID or a COX-2 selective inhibitor while on concomitant aspirin therapy should take a proton pump inhibitor or misoprostol for gastrointestinal protection [5]. Nonacetylated salicylates, such as choline magnesium trisalicylate, or salsalate, are relatively safe and less expensive treatment options that may be considered.

According to Barber and Gibson, safety considerations in the treatment of nonmalignant pain in the elderly recommend against using NSAIDs in light of the evidence that acetaminophen offers similar analgesic benefit with much less associated toxicity [14]. Alternatives should be considered, such as acetaminophen for mild-to-moderate pain and low-dose corticosteroids for inflammatory arthritic conditions. When NSAIDs must be utilized to treat persistent pain in the elderly, they recommend using NSAIDs with a short half-life at the smallest possible dose for the shortest possible duration. Despite this recommendation, they do acknowledge that naproxen, an agent with a half-life of 15 h, has been associated with less cardiovascular risk when compared with the other nonselective NSAIDs and that the long half-life should be a consideration in the prescribing of naproxen [14].

The OARSI guidelines recommend NSAIDs for the treatment of OA of the hip or knee at the lowest effective dose and avoidance of long-term use if possible [35]. In patients with increased GI risk, they recommend a COX-2 selective agent or nonselective NSAID therapy along with a PPI or misoprostol for gastroprotection. They recommend using all NSAIDs with caution in patients with cardiovascular risk factors.

Finally, the most recent AMDA Clinical Practice Guidelines for Pain Management recommend NSAIDs for use if acetaminophen fails to provide relief or if the patient has an acute inflammatory condition [27]. They do note, however, that there is considerable risk of GI bleeding, sodium retention, and renal impairment to occur in the elderly [27]. They also recommend avoiding high doses for prolonged periods of time. For chronic inflammatory states or osteoarthritis, AMDA recommends COX-2 selective inhibitors recognizing that they decrease, but do not eliminate the risk of GI bleeding [27].

Adverse Effects/Precautions

As a class, clearance of NSAID agents from the body differs between younger and older patients [43]. Most NSAIDs undergo both Phase I (oxidation or reduction) and Phase II (glucuronidation or acetylation) metabolism. Phase I metabolism may be reduced in older adults, and deteriorating renal function may prolong exposure to NSAIDs excreted by the kidneys [43]. NSAID toxicity is generally considered to be dose-related; therefore, it would be prudent to start at a low dose and increase slowly, and only as needed.

NSAIDs reduce pain and inflammation by inhibiting the formation of prostaglandins. However, this is also the mechanism for most of the toxicities associated with NSAID therapy, particularly gastrointestinal and renal.

Gastrointestinal Toxicity

NSAID agents cause a host of gastrointestinal (GI) toxicities ranging from dyspepsia, nausea, and diarrhea to mucosal damage such as GI erosions, ulcers, perforations, obstructions, and serious bleeding. Users of nonselective NSAIDs are 3–10 times more likely to have a GI complication than nonusers and this risk increases with age [68]. NSAIDs are responsible for significant morbidity and mortality in the USA: up to 100,000 hospitalizations and 16,000 deaths per year [69, 70]. More recently, a study of ADRs as a cause of hospitalization in older adults 65 years of age and older found that NSAIDs were implicated in 23.5% of the cases [5, 71]. NSAIDs rank among the top five causes of ADRs across all age groups and special consideration should be given to the population of older adults among whom their adverse effects are more pronounced [14]. The decision to begin a patient on NSAID therapy should be one that reflects careful consideration.

Up to 30% of patients complain of dyspepsia on NSAID therapy, which patients may find intolerable [43]. The mechanism leading to this complaint is not clear, and the development of dyspepsia does not correlate to GI mucosal damage [70, 72]. Therapeutic options include lowering the NSAID dose, switching to a different NSAID agent, addition of cytoprotective therapy (such as a proton pump inhibitor), or discontinuing NSAID therapy.

Certainly more worrisome is the development of gastric erosions, perforations, obstructions, and major GI bleeds secondary to NSAID therapy. Approximately 15–30% of NSAID users will show endoscopic evidence of a gastric or duodenal ulcer [72]. The more serious GI events such as perforation, obstruction, or major GI bleed occur in approximately 2% of patients treated with NSAIDs over a year [43]. Risk factors include prior history of a clinical GI event (such as perforation, ulcer, or GI bleed), advanced age (greater than 60 years), concomitant warfarin, antiplatelet or corticosteroid therapy, use of high-dose or multiple NSAIDs, and significant comorbidity [51, 53].

The incidence and severity of these complications illustrate the importance of carefully considering the appropriateness of a patient for NSAID therapy prospectively. Other therapeutic options include concurrent cytoprotective therapy with either misoprostol, a prostaglandin analog, or an antisecretory agent (high dose H2 antagonist or proton pump inhibitor), or use a COX-2-specific NSAID in lieu of a nonspecific NSAID agent. COX-2-specific agents do not afford complete gastroprotection and may still require gastroprotective therapy when used in a population at very high risk for bleeding or concomitantly with aspirin therapy [5]. Studies have suggested that concurrent utilization of a PPI and a COX-2 selective agent decreases GI hospitalization rates in patients older than 75 years of age and in those taking aspirin [56].

Several studies have evaluated the efficacy of concomitant therapies in preventing NSAID-induced mucosal injury. Sucralfate has not shown any benefit in preventing gastric ulcers in NSAID-treated osteoarthritis patients [51]. Recent expert consensus guidelines on reducing GI risks of antiplatelet therapy and NSAID use by the American College of Cardiology Foundation (ACCF) task force recommend against the use of sucralfate for NSAID gastroprotection due to the availability of far-superior alternative agents [51]. Concurrent treatment with an H_2-receptor antagonist has been shown to prevent NSAID-induced duodenal ulcers, but acid suppression at traditional doses was less effective in preventing gastric ulcers [73, 74]. Yeomans et al. demonstrated that omeprazole, a proton-pump inhibitor, was more effective than H_2-receptor antagonists in preventing recurrence of gastroduodenal ulcers [75]. More recently, in a study of elderly aspirin and NSAID users, PPI therapy was found to reduce the risk of GI bleeding in users compared with nonusers, while the use of H_2-receptor antagonists was associated with a significantly higher risk of GI bleeding in users than in nonusers [76]. A meta-analysis of patients receiving NSAIDs showed the H_2-receptor antagonists did not significantly reduce the risk of symptomatic ulcers [77]. PPIs, however, did significantly reduce symptomatic ulcers in this population by 91% [77]. The increasing use of PPI therapy is associated with a decrease in the incidence of peptic ulcers and complications by approximately 40% [77]. Given the burden of a twice daily dosing regimen and the proven superiority of PPI therapy in preventing NSAID-induced ulcer recurrence and overall symptom control, the ACCF guidelines recommend PPIs as preferred therapy [51].

Misoprostol is the only therapy indicated for the prevention of NSAID-related gastrointestinal complications. An oral PGE_1 analog, misoprostol is an antisecretory agent with protective effects on the gastroduodenal mucosa. Silverstein et al. conducted the Misoprostol Ulcer Complication Outcomes Safety Assessment (MUCOSA) study [78]. Concurrent NSAID/misoprostol therapy (200 µg four times daily) resulted in a 40% reduction in the overall rate of complicated upper gastrointestinal events. Misoprostol frequently causes adverse events that can limit therapy in the elderly, such as abdominal pain, heartburn, and diarrhea. Less frequent dosing (such as 200 µg twice daily) results in fewer adverse effects, but research has shown that misoprostol must be taken at least three times daily to effectively prevent NSAID-induced gastric ulcers [79].

Misoprostol has been compared with omeprazole in the healing and prevention of ulcers associated with NSAIDs [80]. Results showed that healing rates in patients with duodenal ulcers were higher in the omeprazole-treated patients, but healing rates in patients with erosions alone were higher with misoprostol. More patients remained ulcer-free when maintained on omeprazole vs. misoprostol, and omeprazole was better tolerated throughout the study. Misoprostol was also more recently shown to be moderately effective at preventing GI bleeds in elderly patients on NSAID therapy, with efficacy less than that of proton pump inhibitors but greater than that of H_2-receptor antagonists [76].

The COX-2-specific NSAID agents have been shown to decrease both endoscopically visualized ulcers and clinically important gastrointestinal events, as compared to nonselective NSAIDs, with a relative risk reduction of 50–65% [81]. Large studies, SUCCESS-1 comparing celecoxib 100 or 200 mg twice daily (vs. diclofenac or naproxen) [66] and CLASS, comparing celecoxib 400 mg twice daily (vs. diclofenac or ibuprofen) [82] showed significantly fewer upper GI events with COX-2 therapy. In the CLASS study, however, the GI ulceration rate increased when the patients were also taking aspirin for cardiovascular prophylaxis [82]. An increase in GI adverse events was not seen in patients on aspirin therapy in the SUCCESS-1 trial, but the study was not powered to determine this endpoint [66]. Subsequent studies have begun to examine the mitigation of COX-2 gastrointestinal safety effects when patients were taking concomitant aspirin therapy, concluding that the gastrointestinal safety benefit is not completely lost but it is markedly diminished [56]. Further studies evaluating the degree of gastrointestinal benefit compared with nonselective NSAID therapy when patients are taking cardioprotective aspirin therapy are required.

Given that two strategies used to reduce the risk of NSAID-induced gastrointestinal toxicities are to add a proton-pump inhibitor to nonselective NSAID therapy or to use a COX-2-specific NSAID instead, it seems reasonable to compare these two strategies in terms of GI outcomes. Chan and colleagues evaluated celecoxib 200 mg twice daily vs. diclofenac 75 mg twice daily plus omeprazole 20 mg for a 6-month period in patients who had used NSAIDs for arthritis and experienced ulcer bleeding [83]. The results showed similar therapeutic outcomes and a similar rate of recurrent bleeding (4.9% of celecoxib-treated patients and 6.4% of diclofenac/omeprazole-treated patients) [83]. Theoretically, one potential advantage to using a COX-2 inhibitor vs. a PPI-NSAID combination may be prevention of lower GI bleeding. COX-2 inhibitors are thought to spare COX-1 prostaglandins throughout the GI tract, but PPIs only block gastric acid production in the upper GI tract. In a study by Goldstein et al. looking at the risk of lower GI ulcers in patients on NSAID therapy, it was found that naproxen plus omeprazole was associated with significantly more breaks in the small intestinal mucosa when compared with celecoxib or placebo [68, 84]. Further data are needed to assess the clinical significance of this finding.

One could argue that the question of whether to use a nonselective NSAID with PPI or misoprostol therapy vs. a COX-2-specific NSAID comes down to economics and tablet burden. However, many patients continue therapy with a PPI despite switching to a COX-2-specific NSAID, negating the cost savings. One incidence in which it may be cost-effective is in a high-risk group, as evidence for coadministration of a PPI with a COX-2 inhibitor resulted in a 50% reduction in upper GI complications [77]. A recent cost-effectiveness analysis of COX-2 selective inhibitors and nonselective NSAIDs alone, or in combination with a PPI, for people with OA was performed in the UK [85]. It was determined that the addition of a PPI to both COX-2 selective inhibitors and nonselective NSAIDs was highly cost effective for all patient groups, even those at low-risk of GI complications [85]. This analysis was sensitive to specific choice of agent, employing the least expensive PPI in all cases, so the authors recommend taking into consideration individual patient cardiovascular and GI risks [85]. As PPIs become available generically and even move to nonprescription status, this may render combination therapy more cost effective. Last, the prescriber must consider the tablet burden for the patient, particularly older patients who may find a twice daily nonselective NSAID plus once daily PPI more burdensome than a once or twice daily COX-2-specific NSAID.

Renal Toxicity, Peripheral Edema, and Hypertension

It has been estimated that approximately 20% of patients taking NSAIDs will develop at least one of a variety of renal function abnormalities [86]. Due to age-related changes, the effects of other drug therapy on renal function (e.g., diuretic-induced volume depletion) and comorbid disease states such as cirrhosis and congestive heart failure, older adults may be at greater risk for renal toxicity from NSAIDs. Examples of NSAID-induced renal toxicity include acute reversible renal failure, impaired renal excretion of water and electrolyte (sodium and potassium), acute interstitial nephritis, and analgesic nephropathy [87].

Renal prostaglandins are involved in the regulation of several homeostatic functions in the kidney including renal blood flow (particularly in cases with decreased actual or effective intravascular volume) and sodium and potassium excretion [43]. It has been shown that the COX-1 isoenzyme is expressed widely throughout the kidney, and it has now been shown that COX-2 is also expressed constitutively in the renal vasculature, glomerulus and ascending limb of the loop of Henle [43]. Consequently, both nonselective and COX-2-specific NSAIDs have been associated with renal dysfunction [88]. Jankovic et al. investigated the incidence of GI bleeding in patients with end stage renal failure on hemodialysis. They found a threefold increase in risk of developing GI bleeding in patients using regular NSAID therapy compared with nonusers [89]. They emphasize the need for effective strategies to prevent GI bleeding in patients on hemodialysis and using NSAIDs. Fluid retention is a more common renal manifestation of NSAID therapy [43]. Although most patients are able to tolerate the enhanced retention of sodium secondary to NSAID therapy, some patients may gain weight, develop peripheral edema, hypertension, and rarely, pulmonary edema [43]. Patients at greater risk for clinical consequences of fluid retention include those with underlying renal disease, congestive heart failure, hepatic insufficiency, or patients receiving diuretics [90]. In the general population of individuals greater than 55 years of age, there was a twofold increase in the risk of hospitalization from congestive heart failure with the addition of an NSAID to a diuretic regimen [86]. Additionally, there is a tenfold increase in the risk of hospitalization in individuals with a previous diagnosis of CHF when an NSAID is added [86]. Body weight for at risk patients should be monitored carefully, particularly after initiating or increasing NSAID therapy.

It is not uncommon to find older adults taking both an NSAID agent and an antihypertensive agent. In one study, approximately 52% of elderly (over 60 years of age) had diagnosed or untreated hypertension, and 12–15% of elderly were receiving at least one NSAID agent and an antihypertensive agent concurrently [91]. Gurwitz et al. found that older adults (over 65 years of age) are 1.7-fold more likely to require initiation of an antihypertensive agent when also taking an NSAID agent than patients who are not taking an NSAID agent [91]. Patients at greater risk for blood pressure changes with concomitant use of an antihypertensive agent and an NSAID include those patients with congestive heart failure, liver disease, or kidney disease [86]. Meta-analyses of the effect of NSAID therapy on blood pressure show a clinically significant mean increase of 5.0 mmHg, particularly in patients with controlled hypertension [92, 93]. Of those nonselective NSAIDs assessed, indomethacin, naproxen, ibuprofen, and piroxicam produced the greatest increase in mean blood pressure [94, 95]. Antihypertensive agents, with the exception of calcium channel blockers and angiotensin II receptor antagonists, act on prostaglandin synthesis and so, the degree to which a particular NSAID inhibits prostaglandin production is proportional to the degree that it affects hypertension control [86]. NSAIDs may antagonize the antihypertensive effects of beta blockers, ACE inhibitors, and diuretics [86].

COX-2-specific NSAIDs have also been associated with an increase in blood pressure [86, 96]. Whelton et al. specifically evaluated the effects of celecoxib 200 mg/day and rofecoxib 25 mg/day on blood pressure and edema in patients 65 years and older with systemic hypertension and osteoarthritis [97]. Both agents lead to an increased systolic blood pressure (change >20 mmHg plus absolute value ≥140 mmHg). The study design prohibited a legitimate comparison between agents, however, since the study dose of rofecoxib (25 mg) is not considered to be equianalgesic to the dosing of celecoxib (200 mg each day) [98]. The article finally published by Whelton et al. nonetheless reported a 6.9% incidence of hypertension and a 4.7% incidence of significant new-onset or worsening edema associated with weight gain within the celecoxib treatment group [99].

Collins et al. showed that a sustained increase (over a few years) in diastolic blood pressure of 5–6 mmHg may be associated with a 67% increase in total stroke occurrence and a 15% increase in coronary heart disease events [96, 99]. In a review of NSAID-induced hypertension, Johnson suggests that is critical to determine whether an older patient even requires NSAID therapy, when perhaps non-pharmacologic interventions or other analgesics may suffice [99]. Should the patient require NSAID therapy, the patient should be evaluated carefully for increases in blood pressure, edema, and weight gain [99].

Cardiovascular Disease and Thrombosis

Aspirin (a strong COX-1 inhibitor) has been widely accepted as a therapeutic intervention shown to prevent cardiovascular and cerebrovascular disease due to its ability to irreversibly inhibit platelet aggregation [100]. Nonselective NSAIDs reversibly inhibit platelet aggregation, but concern has arisen that COX-2 selective NSAIDs that lack COX-1 inhibition may lead to an increased incidence of thrombosis in patients who are at risk. In the VIGOR trial (rofecoxib 50 mg/day vs. naproxen 1,000 mg/day), there was a statistically significant decrease in nonfatal myocardial infarctions in the naproxen-treated group [101]. Patients in this study were not permitted to take low-dose aspirin for cardiovascular purposes; therefore, it is unclear whether this observed effect was due to cardioprotection provided by naproxen therapy or due to a prothrombotic effect of rofecoxib. Nor are we able to draw conclusions from the large CLASS trial, in which celecoxib was compared with nonselective NSAIDs [82]. Patients in the CLASS trial were allowed to take low-dose aspirin, and the incidence of nonfatal myocardial infarctions was similar in the celecoxib-treated patients and the ibuprofen or diclofenac-treated patients [82]. Based on a meta-analysis of COX-2 agents, rofecoxib and valdecoxib were removed from the market for increased risk of myocardial infarction and cardiovascular events. The American Heart Association recommends acetaminophen, non-acetylated salicylates, and short-term opioids instead of NSAIDs and COX-2 inhibitor agents in patients with coronary artery disease [3].

   In addition to the concern about increased risk of GI events when COX-2 selective agents are used with low-dose aspirin, there also is concern about the deleterious effect of some traditional NSAIDs on the cardioprotection afforded by low-dose aspirin. In a recent study by Gladding et al., the antiplatelet effects of selected NSAID agents were analyzed ex vivo to determine their potential to antagonize the antiplatelet effect of aspirin [102]. In this study, the NSAID was given 2 h prior to aspirin 300 mg in normal healthy volunteers and analyzed 12 h after NSAID administration. It was determined that indomethacin, naproxen, and ibuprofen significantly antagonize the antiplatelet effect of aspirin, while celecoxib and sulindac did not have the same deleterious effect [102]. The authors concluded that of the NSAIDs evaluated, celecoxib and sulindac may be the agents of choice for patients requiring aspirin therapy and NSAIDs [102]. According to a warning put out by the FDA in 2006, if a patient is taking a daily aspirin and ibuprofen 400 mg, the aspirin should be administered 30 min prior to the ibuprofen or no less than 8 h after an ibuprofen dose, to eliminate competitive drug interactions for the inhibition of cyclooxygenase [103]. According to the AGS guidelines for the management of pain in older adults, patients taking aspirin for cardioprotection should not use ibuprofen [5].

Summary

In summary, clinicians need to carefully consider whether NSAID therapy is appropriate for any given older adult, given the pathogenesis of their pain, and risk factors for NSAID-induced adverse effects. At equipotent doses, the efficacy of all NSAIDs (COX-2 selective or nonselective) is similar, but individual patients may respond better to one agent than another. Additional considerations when selecting an NSAID include adverse effects (particularly gastrointestinal and renal), dosing frequency, patient preference, and cost. For patients at risk for gastrotoxicity, consider a COX-2 selective NSAID or a nonselective NSAID in combination with a proton-pump inhibitor or misoprostol. Patients at high risk for GI bleeding may require the addition of a PPI to a COX-2 selective inhibitor. Patients taking NSAID agents should be carefully monitored for adverse effects, particularly GI dyspepsia and bleeding, weight gain, fluid retention, and hypertension. Patients at risk for cardiovascular or cerebrovascular disease should receive low-dose aspirin in combination with NSAID therapy. Attention should be given to the dosing schedule of the nonselective NSAID in respect to the aspirin. In this setting, one may wish to consider naproxen until more data become available.

Conclusion

There are a variety of oral agents available to assist in the challenge of pain relief. Additionally, some nonopioid topical agents include capsaicin, aspirin or NSAID-based creams, and lidocaine-based creams [21]. For certain types of pain, other nonopioid agents should be considered as well, e.g., bisphosphonates for pain associated with skeletal metastasis (see Chap. 8) [103–105].

It is important to note that oftentimes, even in older adults, more than one nonopioid medication may be necessary to control pain. When pain persists after adequate trials of nonopioid agents and their combinations, opioid interventions should be considered. The next chapter deals with the use of opioids and adjuvant medications in depth.

References

1. Shimp LA. Safety issues in the pharmacologic management of chronic pain in the elderly. Pharmacotherapy. 1998;18(6):1313–22.
2. Fine PG. Chronic pain management in older adults: special considerations. J Pain Symptom Manage. 2009;38:S4–14.
3. Kroenke K, Krebs EE, Bair MJ. Pharmacotherapy of chronic pain: a synthesis of recommendations from systematic reviews. Gen Hosp Psychiatry. 2009;31:206–19.
4. Latham J, Davis BD. The socioeconomic impact of chronic pain. Disabil Rehabil. 1994;16:39–44.
5. AGS Panel on the Pharmacological Management of Persistent Pain in Older Persons. Pharmacological management of persistent pain in older persons. J Am Geriatr Soc. 2009;57:1331–46.
6. Crook J, Rodeout E, Browne G. The prevalence of pain complaints in a general population. Pain. 1984;18:299–314.
7. Workman BS, Ciccone V, Christophidis N. Pain management for the elderly. Aust Fam Physician. 1989;18:1515–27.
8. Ferrell BA. Pain management in elderly people. J Am Geriatr Soc. 1991;39:64–73.
9. Pitkala K, Standberg T, Tilvis R. Management of nonmalignant pain in home-dwelling older people: a population-based survey. J Am Geriatr Soc. 2002;50:1861–5.

10. Landi F, Onder G, Cesari M, et.al. Pain management in frail, community-living elderly patients. Arch Intern Med. 2001;161:2721–4.
11. Cramer GW, Galer BS, Mendelson MA, Thompson GD. A drug use evaluation of selected opioid and nonopioid analgesics in the nursing facility setting. J Am Geriatr Soc. 2000;48(4). http://www.mdconsult.com.
12. Cavalieri T. Pain management in the elderly. J Am Osteopath Assoc. 2002;102:481–5.
13. Beyth R, Shorr R. Epidemiology of adverse drug reactions in the elderly by drug class. Drugs Aging. 1999;14(3):231–9.
14. Barber JB, Gibson SJ. Treatment of chronic non-malignant pain in the elderly: safety considerations. Drug Saf. 2009;32:(6):457–74.
15. Karp JF, Shega JW, Morone NE, Weiner DK. Advances in understanding the mechanisms and management of persistent pain in older adults. Br J Anaesth. 2008;101:111–20.
16. Pasero C, Rred B, McCaffery M. Pain in the elderly. In: McCaffery M, Pasero C, editors. Pain clinical manual. 2nd ed. St. Louis: Mosby; 1999. p. 674–710.
17. Davis MP, Srivastava M. Demographics, assessment and management of pain in the elderly. Drugs Aging. 2003;20(1):23–57.
18. Kaiko RF. Age and morphine analgesia in cancer patients with postoperative pain. Clin Pharmacol Ther. 1980;28:823–6.
19. Bellville JW, Forrest WH Jr, Miller E, Brown BW Jr. Influence of age on pain relief from analgesics. A study of postoperative patients. JAMA. 1971;217:1835–41.
20. Beers MH. Age-related changes as a risk factor for medication-related problems. Generations (Winter). 2000–2001;24(4):22–7. http://www.generationsjournal.org. Accessed 17 Nov 2009.
21. Gloth FM. Pain management in older adults: prevention and treatment. J Am Geriatr Soc. 2001;49:188–99.
22. Furst DE, Munster T. Nonsteroidal anti-inflammatory drugs, disease-modifying antirheumatic drugs, nonopioid analgesics, and drugs used in gout. In: Katzung BG, editor. Basic and clinical pharmacology. 8th ed. New York: McGraw Hill; 2001. p. 615.
23. Graham GG, Scott KF. Mechanism of action of paracetamol. Am J Ther. 2005;12:46–55.
24. Chandrasekharan NV, Dai H, Turepu Roos KL, Evanson NK, Tomsik J, Elton TS, et al. COX-3, a cyclooxygenase-1 variant inhibited by acetaminophen and other analgesic/antipyretic drugs: cloning, structure, and expression. Proc Natl Acad Sci USA. 2002;9921:13926–31.
25. Kis B, Snipes JA, Busija DW. Acetaminophen and the cyclooxygenase-3 puzzle: sorting out the facts, fictions, and uncertainties. J Pharmacol Exp Ther. 2005;315:1–7.
26. McEvoy GK, editor. AHFS drug information. Bethesda: American Society of Health-System Pharmacists; 2002. p. 2099.
27. American Medical Directors Association. Pain management clinical practice guideline. Columbia, MD: American Medical Directors Association; 2009.
28. Amadio P Jr, Cummings DM. Evaluation of acetaminophen in the management of osteoarthritis of the knee. Curr Ther Res. 1983;34:59–66.
29. Bradley JD, Brandt KD, Katz BP, Kalasinski LA, Ryan SI. Comparison of an anti-inflammatory dose of ibuprofen, an analgesic dose of ibuprofen, and acetaminophen in the treatment of patient with osteoarthritis of the knee. N Engl J Med. 1991;325:87–91.
30. Williams HJ, Ward JR, Egger MJ, Neuner R, Brooks RH, Clegg DO, et al. Comparison of naproxen and acetaminophen in a two-year study of treatment of osteoarthritis of the knee. Arthritis Rheum. 1993;9:1196–206.
31. Towheed T, Maxwell L, Judd M, Catton M, Hochberg MC, Wells GA. Acetaminophen for osteoarthritis. Cochrane Database Syst Rev. 2006;Issue 1. Art. No.: CD004257. DOI:10.1002/14651858.CD004257.pub2.
32. Lee C, Straus WL, Balshaw R, Barlas S, Vogel S, Schnitzer TJ. A comparison of the efficacy and safety of nonsteroidal anti-inflammatory agents versus acetaminophen in the treatment of osteoarthritis: a meta-analysis. Arthritis Rheum. 2004;51(5):746–54.
33. American College of Rheumatology Subcommittee on Osteoarthritis Guidelines. Recommendations for the medical management of osteoarthritis of the hip and knee. Arthritis Rheum. 2002;43:1905–15.

34. American Pain Society. Guideline for the management of pain in osteoarthritis, rheumatoid arthritis, and juvenile chronic arthritis. 2nd ed. Glenview: American Pain Society; 2002.

35. OARSI recommendations for the management of hip and knee osteoarthritis. Part II: OARSI evidence-based, expert consensus guidelines. Osteoarthritis Cartilage. 2008;16:137–62.

36. Clissold SP. Paracetamol and phenacetin. Drugs. 1986;32 Suppl 4:46–59.

37. Shamoon M, Hochberg MC. The role of acetaminophen in the management of patients with osteoarthritis. Am J Med. 2001;110(3A):46S–49.

38. Bannwarth B, Fehourcq F, Lagrange F, Matoga M, Maury S, Palisson M, et al. Single and multiple dose pharmacokinetics of acetaminophen (paracetamol) in polymedicated very old patients with rheumatic pain. J Rheumatol. 2001;28(1):182–4.

39. Sandler DP, Smith JC, Weinberg CR, Buckalew VM, Dennis VW, Blythe WB, et al. Analgesic use and chronic renal disease. N Engl J Med. 1989;320:1238–43.

40. Perneger TV, Whelton PK, Klag MJ. Risk of kidney failure associated with the use of acetaminophen, aspirin, and nonsteroidal anti-inflammatory drugs. N Engl J Med. 1994;331:1675–9.

41. Henrich WL, Agodaoa LE, Barrett B, Bennett WM, Blantz RC, Buckalew VM, et al. Analgesics and the kidney: summary and recommendations to the Scientific Advisory Board of the national Kidney Foundation from an Ad Hoc Committee of the National Kidney Foundation. Am J Kidney Dis. 1996;27:162–5.

42. National Kidney Foundation. Analgesics. http://www.kidney.org/general/atoz/content/analgesics.html. Accessed 2 Feb 2003.

43. Whitcomb DC, Block GD. Association of acetaminophen hepatotoxicity with fasting and ethanol use. JAMA. 1994;273:1845–50.

44. Schiodt FV, Rochling FA, Casey DL, Lee WM. Acetaminophen toxicity in an urban county hospital. N Engl J Med. 1997;337:1112–7.

45. Health News Daily. OTC acetaminophen labeling should warn about liver damage risk from higher-than-recommended doses – NDAC members. September 20 2002;14(183). http://128.121.3.174/NR/FDC/FDCViewerIncludes/frameset.asp?targetGUID= {AACA1D0F-A5EE-48E9-9FAF-000E4D313FA2}&PopupWidth=730&PopupHeight=680. Accessed 2 Feb 2003.

46. Cham E, Hall L, Ernst AA, Weiss SJ. Awareness and use of over-the-counter pain medications: a survey of emergency department patients. South Med J. 2002;95:529–35.

47. Herr K, Bjoro K, Steffensmeier J, Rakel B. The Guidelines for the Acute Pain Management in Older Adults. University of Iowa. 2006 http://www.guideline.gov/summary/summary. aspx?doc_id=10198&nbr=00538. Accessed 11 Sept 2009.

48. Baker DE. Acetaminophen: is it time for a change in utilization to decrease the risk of hepatotoxicity. Hosp Pharm. 2009;44:843–5.

49. Parra D, Beckey NP, Stevens GR. The effect of acetaminophen on the international normalized ratio in patients stabilized on warfarin therapy. Pharmacotherapy. 2007;27(5): 675–83.

50. Stillman MJ, Stillman MT. Appropriate use of NSAIDs: considering cardiovascular risk in the elderly. Geriatrics. 2007;62:16–21.

51. Bhatt DL, Scheiman J, Abraham NS, Antman EM, Chan FKL, Furberg CD, Johnson DA, Mahaffey KW, Quigley EM. ACCF/ACG/AHA 2008 expert consensus document on reducing the gastrointestinal risks of antiplatelet therapy and NSAID use: a report of the American College of Cardiology Foundation Task Force on Clinical Expert Consensus Documents. Circulation. 2008;118:1894–909.

52. Ebgert A. Postoperative pain management in the frail and elderly. Clin Geriatr Med. 1996;12(Part 3):583.

53. Bell GM, Schnitzer TJ. Cox-2 inhibitors and other nonsteroidal anti-inflammatory drugs in the treatment of pain in the elderly. Clin Geriatr Med. 2001;17:489–502.

54. Roberts LJ II, Morrow JD. Analgesic-antipyretic and anti-inflammatory agents and drugs employed in the treatment of gout. In: Hardman JG, Limbird LE, editors. Goodman and Gilman's the pharmacologic basis of therapeutics. 10th ed. New York: McGraw-Hill; 2001. p. 687–92.

55. APhA Special Report. Emerging therapies for inflammation and pain: the role of cyclooxygenase selectivity. Washington, DC: APhA; 1999. p. 1–19.
56. APhA Special Report. Therapeutic advances in the management of pain: the role of cyclooxygenase-2-specific inhibitors. Washington, DC: APhA; 2002. p. 1–21.
57. McGettigan P, Henry D. Cardiovascular risk and inhibition of cyclooxygenase: a systematic review of the observational studies of selective and nonselective inhibitors of cyclooxygenase 2. JAMA. 2006;296(13):1633–44.
58. Carr DB, Jacox AK, Chapman CR, Ferrell B, Fields HL, Heidrich G, et al. Acute pain management: operative or medical procedures and trauma. Clinical Practice Guideline No. 1. AHCPR Pub. No. 92-0032. Rockville, MD: Agency for Health Care Policy and Research, Publich Health Service, U.S. Department of Health and Human Services; 1992.
59. Dahl V, Raeder JC. Non-opioid postoperative analgesia. Acta Anaesthesiol Scand. 2000;44:1191–203.
60. Varrassi G, Panella L, Piroli A, Marinangeli F, Varrassi S, Wolman I, et al. The effects of perioperative ketorolac infusion on postoperative pain and endocrine-metabolic response. Anesth Analg. 1994;78:514–9.
61. Cheung R, Krishnaswarmi S, Kowalski K. Analgesic efficacy of celecoxib in postoperative oral surgery pain: a single-dose, two-center, randomized, double-blind, active- and placebo-controlled study. Clin Ther. 2007;29:2498–510.
62. Derry S, Barden J, McQuay HJ, Moore RA. Single dose oral celecoxib for acute postoperative pain in adults. Cochrane Database Syst Rev. 2008;Issue 4. Art.No: CD004233. doi:10.1002/14651858.CD004233.pub2.
63. Myers SL, Brandt KD, Ehlich JW, Braunstein EM, Shelbourne KD, Heck DA, Kalasinski LA. Synovial inflammation in patients with early osteoarthritis of the knee. J Rheumatol. 1990;17:1662–9.
64. Ryu J, Treadwell BV, Mankin HJ. Biochemical and metabolic abnormalities in normal and osteoarthritis human articular cartilage. Arthritis Rheum. 1984;27(1):49–57.
65. Brandt KD. Toward pharmacologic modification of joint damage in osteoarthritis (editorial). Ann Intern Med. 1995;122(1):874–5.
66. Singh G, Fort JG, Goldstein JL, Levy RA, Hanrahan PS, Bello AE, et al. Celecoxib versus naproxen and diclofenac in osteoarthritis patients: SUCCESS-I study. Am J Med. 2006;119:255–66.
67. Altman RD. Practical considerations for the pharmacologic management of osteoarthritis. Am J Manag Care. 2009;15:S236–43.
68. Stillman MJ, Stillman MT. Choosing nonselective NSAIDs and selective COX-2 inhibitors in the elderly: a clinical use pathway. Geriatrics. 2007;62:26–34.
69. Singh G. Recent considerations in nonsteroidal anti-inflammatory drug gastropathy. Am J Med. 1998;105 Suppl 1B:31S.
70. Wolfe M Lichtenstein D, Singh G. Gastrointestinal toxicity of nonsteroidal anti-inflammatory drugs. N Engl J Med. 1999;34:1888–99.
71. Fransechi M, Scarcelli C, Niro V, Seripa D, Pazienza AM, Colusso AM, et al. Prevalence, clinical features and avoidability of adverse reactions as a cause of admission to a geriatric unit: a prospective study of 1756 patients. Drug Saf. 2008;32:545–56.
72. Laine L. Nonsteroidal anti-inflammatory drug gastropathy. Gastrointest Endosc Clin N Am. 1996;6(Part 3):489.
73. Robinson MG, Griffin JW Jr, Bowers J, Kogan FJ, Kogut DG, Lanza FL, et al. Effect of ranitidine on gastroduodenal mucosal damage induced by nonsteroidal anti-inflammatory drugs. Dig Dis Sci. 1989;34:424–8.
74. Ehsanullah RSB, Page MC, Tildesley G, et al. Prevention of gastrointestinal damage induced by non-steroidal anti-inflammatory drugs: controlled trial of ranitidine. BMJ 1988;297: 1017–21.
75. Yeomans ND, Tulassay Z, Juhasz L, et al. A comparison of omeprazole with ranitidine for ulcers associated with nonsteroidal anti-inflammatory drugs. N Engl J Med. 1998;338: 719–26.

76. Pilotto A, Franceschi M, Leandro G, Paris F, Niro V, Longo MG, et al. The risk of upper gastrointestinal bleeding in elderly users of aspirin and other non-steroidal anti-inflammatory drugs: the role of gastroprotective drugs. Aging Clin Exp Res. 2003;15(6):494–9.
77. Lanas A, Ferrandez A. NSAID-induced gastrointestinal damage: current clinical management and recommendations for prevention. Chin J Dig Dis. 2006;7:127–33.
78. Silverstein FE, Graham DY, Senior JR, Davies HW, Struthers BJ, Bittman RM et al. Misoprostol reduces serious gastrointestinal complications in patients with rheumatoid arthritis receiving nonsteroidal anti-inflammatory drugs: a randomized, double-blind, placebo-controlled trial. Ann Intern Med. 1995;123:241–9.
79. Raskin JB, White RH, Jackson JE, et al. Misoprostol dosage in the prevention of nonsteroidal anti-inflammatory drug-induced gastric and duodenal ulcers: a comparison of three regimens. Ann Intern Med. 1995;123:344–50.
80. Hawkey CJ, Karrasch JA, Szczepanski L, Walker DG, Barkun A, Swannell AJ, et al. Omeprazole compared with misoprostol for ulcers associated with nonsteroidal anti-inflammatory drugs. N Engl J Med. 1998;338:727–34.
81. Laine L. Approaches to nonsteroidal anti-inflammatory drug use in the high-risk patient. Gastroenterology. 2001;120:594–606.
82. Silverstein FE, Faich G, Goldsterin JL, et al. Gastrointestinal toxicity with celecoxib vs. nonsteroidal anti-inflammatory drugs for osteoarthritis and rheumatoid arthritis: the CLASS study: a randomized controlled trial. Celecoxib Long-term Arthritis Safety Study. J Am Med Assoc. 2000;284(10):1247–55.
83. Chan FKL, Hung LCT, Suen BY, et al. Celecoxib versus diclofenac and omperazole in reducing the risk of recurrent ulcer bleeding in patients with arthritis. N Engl J Med. 2002;347:2104–10.
84. Goldstein JL, Eisen G, Lewis B, et al. Celecoxib is associated with devar small bowel lesions than naproxen and omeprazole in healthy subjects as determined by capsule endoscopy (abstract). Am J Gastroenterol. 2003;98:S297
85. Latimer N, Lord J, Grant RL, O'Mahony R, Dickson J, Conaghan PG, et al. Cost effectiveness of COX2 selective inhibitors and traditional NSAIDs alone or in combination with a proton pump inhibitor for people with osteoarthritis. BMJ. 2009;339:b2538.
86. Whelton A. Clinical implications of nonopioid analgesia for relief of mild-to-moderate pain in patients with or at risk for cardiovascular disease. Am J Cardiol. 2006;97 Suppl:3E–9E.
87. Schlondorff D. Renal complications of nonsteroidal anti-inflammatory drugs. Kidney Int. 1993;44:643–53.
88. Morales E, Mucksavage JJ. Pharmacotherapy. 2002;22:1317–21.
89. Jankovic SM, Aleksic J, Rakovic S, Aleksic A, Stevanovic I, Stefanovic-Stoimenov N, et al. Nonsteroidal anti-inflammatory drugs and risk of gastrointestinal bleeding among patients on hemodialysis (abstract). J Nephrol. 2009;22(4):502–7.
90. Brater D. Effects of nonsteroidal anti-inflammatory drugs on renal function: focus on cyclooxygenase-2-selective inhibition. Am J Med. 1999;107 Suppl 6A:65S.
91. Gurwitz JH, Avorn J, Bohn RL, Glynn RJ, Monane M, Mogun H, et al. Initiation of antihypertensive treatment during nonsteroidal anti-inflammatory drug therapy. JAMA. 1994;272:781–6.
92. Johnson AG, Nguyen TV, Day RO. Do nonsteroidal anti-inflammatory drugs affect blood pressure? A meta-analysis. Ann Intern Med. 1994;121:289–300.
93. Pope JE, Anderson JJ, Felson DT. A meta-analysis of the effects of nonsteroidal anti-inflammatory drugs on blood pressure. Arch Intern Med. 1993;153:477–84.
94. LeLorier J, Bombardier C, Burgess E, Moist L, Wright N, Cartier P, et al. Practical considerations for the use of nonsteroidal anti-inflammatory drugs and cyclo-oxygenase-2 inhibitors in hypertension and kidney disease. Can J Cardiol. 2002;18:1301–8.
95. Cheng HF, Harris RC. Does cyclooxygenase-2 affect blood pressure? Curr Hypertens Rep. 2003;5:87–92.
96. Collins R, Peto R, MacMahon S, Hebert P, Fiebach NH, Eberlein KA, et al. Epidemiology. Blood pressure, stroke and coronary heart disease. Part 2, short-term reductions in blood

pressure: overview of randomized drug trials in their epidemiological context. Lancet. 1990;335:827–38.

97. Whelton A, White WB, Bello AE, Puma JA, Fort JG, SUCCESS-VII Investigators. Effects of celecoxib and rofecoxib on blood pressure and edema in patients > or = 65 years of age with systemic hypertension and osteoarthritis. Am J Cardiol. 2002;90:959–63.

98. Geba GP, Weaver AL, Polis AB, Dixon ME, Schnitzer TJ. Efficacy of rofecoxib, celecoxib, and acetaminophen in osteoarthritis of the knee. JAMA 2002;287:64–71.

99. Johnson AG. NSAIDs and blood pressure: clinical importance for older patients. Drugs Aging. 1998;12:17–27.

100. Hennekens C. Update on aspirin in the treatment and prevention of cardiovascular disease. Am Heart J. 1999;137:S9.

101. Bombardier D, Laine L, Reicin A, Shapiro D, Burgos-Vargas R, Davis B, et al. Comparison of upper gastrointestinal toxicity of rofecoxib and naproxen in patients with rheumatoid arthritis. VIGOR Study Group. N Eng J Med. 2000;343:1520–8.

102. Gladding PA, Webster MWI, Farrell HB, Zeng IS, Park R, Ruijne N. The antiplatelet effect of six non-steroidal anti-inflammatory drugs and their pharmacodynamic interaction with aspirin in healthy volunteers. Am J Cardiol. 2008;101:1060–3.

103. Gloth FM III. Pain management in older adults: prevention and treatment. J Am Geriatr Soc. 2001;49:188–99.

104. Gloth FM III. The use of a bisphosphonate (etidronate) to improve metastatic bone pain in three hospice patients. Clin J Pain. 1995;11:333–5.

105. Hortobagyi GN, Theriault RL, Lester P, Blayney D, Lipton A, Sinoff C, et al. Pamidronate in reducing skeletal complications in patients with breast cancer and lytic bone metastases. Protocol 19 Aredia Breast Cancer Study Group. N Engl J Med. 1996;335:1785–91.

Chapter 8
Pharmacotherapy of Pain in Older Adults: Opioid and Adjuvant

Mary Lynn McPherson and Tanya J. Uritsky

Remember how much you do not know. Do not pour strange medicines into your patients.

Sir William Osler

Opioids

Mechanism of Action

Opioids are naturally occurring, semisynthetic, and synthetic drugs whose effects are mediated through opioid receptors, altering the perception and emotional response to painful stimuli [1, 2]. There are three major classes of opioid receptors: μ (mu), κ (kappa), and δ (delta), with subtypes within each receptor class [3]. Opioid receptors are found in the periaqueductal grey matter and throughout the spinal cord, as well as nonneural sites such as joint synovium and intestinal mucosa [1, 2].

The analgesic effects of opioids are primarily attributed to the activation of the μ and κ receptors. Additional effects from μ-receptor stimulation include respiratory depression, miosis, euphoria, and reduced gastrointestinal mobility. Stimulation of the κ receptor causes dysphoria, psychotomimetic effects, miosis, and respiratory depression in addition to analgesia [3].

Opioid analgesics can be further categorized based on the type of interaction, they have with opioid receptors, including receptor affinity (how tightly the opioid binds to the receptor) and intrinsic activity (amount of receptor stimulation) [5]. These categories include opioid agonists, partial agonists, agonist–antagonists, and antagonists.

M.L. McPherson (✉)
Department of Pharmacy Practice and Science, University of Maryland School of Pharmacy, 20 N. Pine Street, Room 405, Baltimore, Maryland 21201, USA
e-mail: mmcphers@rx.umaryland.edu

F.M. Gloth, III (ed.), *Handbook of Pain Relief in Older Adults: An Evidence-Based Approach*, Aging Medicine, DOI 10.1007/978-1-60761-618-4_8,
© Springer Science+Business Media, LLC 2011

Pure opioid agonists (such as morphine) bind to an opioid receptor, which causes intracellular changes resulting in analgesia. There is no obvious "ceiling" effect with a pure opioid agonist, and the dosage may be increased as needed until either analgesia is achieved or adverse effects occur.

Partial opioid agonists (such as buprenorphine) bind to the receptor, but with less intrinsic activity. Partial opioid agonists may exhibit a "ceiling" effect, where dosage increases will not result in additional analgesia. Concurrent administration of a pure opioid agonist and a partial opioid agonist may result in the displacement of the pure opioid agent from the receptor, which may lessen the analgesia or cause opioid withdrawal [1].

Mixed agonist–antagonist opioids (such as pentazocine) produce agonist effects at one receptor and antagonist effects at another. For example, pentazocine is an agonist at κ receptors, causing analgesia as well as psychotomimetic effects, and serves as a weak μ-receptor antagonist. When a mixed agonist–antagonist is administered with a pure opioid agonist, the antagonist effects at the μ receptor can cause an acute withdrawal syndrome [1].

An opioid antagonist (such as naloxone) binds to the receptor but causes no physiologic response. Opioid antagonists block the pharmacologic effects of opioid agonists and may be used clinically to treat an overdose situation caused by an opioid agonist.

Place in Therapy

Opioid analgesics are used to treat moderate-to-severe pain. They are effective in the treatment of all types of pain, including acute pain from surgery or trauma, and chronic cancer and noncancer pain.

The AHCPR guidelines entitled, "Acute Pain Management: Operative or Medical Procedures and Trauma" advocate for the use of opioids as initial analgesic therapy in the management of moderately severe-to-severe pain [4, 5]. NSAID agents may be used concurrently with opioids to decrease levels of inflammatory mediators generated at the site of tissue injury and to allow the reduction of opioid dosing (and subsequent opioid-induced adverse effects). Opioids should be dosed around the clock during the time period patients are likely to require an opioid (e.g., 48 h following surgery) instead of "as needed." Alternately, patient controlled analgesia (PCA) is a safe and effective method of providing opioid therapy for postoperative pain control. With PCA therapy, the patient is able to activate a bolus dose of parenteral opioid as needed. A low-dose basal infusion of opioid may be added at night to allow uninterrupted sleep. Patients should switch to oral opioid therapy as soon as possible.

The AHCPR guidelines recognize the effectiveness of opioids in older adults with acute pain [4]. Caution should be used in opioid dosing in older adults because they may be more sensitive to the analgesic effects (i.e., higher peak drug concentration and longer duration of pain relief) and adverse effects (i.e., sedation, respiratory depression). Because older adults have an increased fat-to-lean body mass ratio and reduced renal function, opioid selection becomes an important issue. For example, some opioids cause cognitive and neuropsychiatric dysfunction (i.e., normeperidine [metabolite of meperidine] or morphine-6-glucuronide [metabolite of morphine]) and should be dosed cautiously or avoided.

The Clinical Guidelines for the Use of Chronic Opioid Therapy in Chronic Noncancer pain provide guidance on appropriate utilization of opioids in noncancer pain [6]. The expert panel recommends that initial treatment with opioids be considered a trial and that opioid selection, dosing and titration should be individualized according to the individual patient's situation (past exposure, health status, etc.). They emphasize that frail older adults and patients with multiple comorbidities may benefit from more cautious titration of therapy. No one opioid has been proven more effective than another as initial therapy. Evidence is not sufficient to recommend the use of short-acting versus long-acting opioids or as-needed versus around-the-clock dosing. The proposed benefits of transitioning to long-acting opioids include the need for consistent pain control, improved adherence and lower risk of misuse or abuse [6]. Breakthrough pain medication should be considered on a risk-versus-benefit analysis. The panel stresses the need to reassess patients for change in pain intensity, progress toward therapeutic goals, presence of adverse effects, and adherence to therapy [6].

The World Health Organization analgesic ladder is an effective, validated model for the treatment of mild, moderate, and severe pain [7, 8]. In this model, nonopioids are used as step 1 agents for mild pain. Steps 2 recommends "weak" opioids such as codeine or tramadol, and step 3 recommends strong opioids such as morphine, oxycodone, hydromorphone, fentanyl, or methadone (possibly in combination with nonopioids) to treat persisting or increasing pain [9]. In all cases, an adjuvant agent can be utilized [7]. Additionally, it may be appropriate to try different nonopioid agents or combinations of agents before moving up the ladder. This approach of administering the right drug, in the right dose, at the right time is inexpensive and is 80–90% effective [7]. In cancer pain, there has been a suggestion to transform the ladder more into the concept of an elevator, as many patients present with severe pain and utilization of strong opioids may be delayed by the untrained clinicians simply following the ladder [9]. This approach would allow the clinician to take the "elevator" to the appropriate floor rather than climbing the rungs of a ladder [9].

Mercadente and Arcuri make more specific recommendations for the utilization of opioids in cancer pain in the elderly based on the steps of the WHO ladder [10]. They recommend beginning opioid therapy when elderly patients have specific contraindications or intolerances to nonopioid therapies. Instead of weak opioids, such as codeine and propoxyphene, for moderate pain, they recommend low doses of strong opioids such as morphine and oxycodone. For older adults with severe pain, they recommend starting strong opioid therapy immediately without delaying for trials of milder analgesics. Drug selection should be based on the duration of action, route of administration, adverse effect potential, and response to therapy. Propoxyphene, codeine, and meperidine are recognized as nonpreferred agents [10].

Opioids are also used in the management of neuropathic pain, such as diabetic neuropathy and postherpetic neuralgia (PHN). The International Association for the Study of Pain (IASP) recommends opioids as second-line therapies in the treatment of neuropathic pain, second to secondary amine tricyclic antidepressants (TCAs) and selective serotonin/norepinephrine reuptake inhibitor antidepressants, gabapentin and pregabalin, and topical lidocaine [11]. Opioids, although having demonstrated efficacy in multiple randomized controlled clinical trials, are second-line due to the incidence and persistence of significant side effects, the risk for abuse and diversion and the existence of better tolerated and potentially less risky therapeutic options [11]. Opioids are therefore recommended for patients who fail to respond to or cannot tolerate first-line recommendations [11].

The American Pain Society guidelines for the management of pain in arthritis recommend that opioids be used for patients with OA and RA when other medications and nonpharmacologic interventions fail to produce adequate pain relief, and the patient's quality of life is adversely affected by the pain [12]. Morphine, oxycodone, hydrocodone, or other mu-opioid agonists are recommended, possibly concurrently with a nonopioid agent. Codeine is not recommended due to mixed results regarding therapeutic efficacy, but even more important is the high incidence of adverse effects associated with codeine therapy.

Oxycodone has been shown to be effective in treating OA pain, using both immediate-release tablets and long-acting tablets. In a study by Roth et al., oxycodone 10 mg controlled-release tablets produced 19–53% improvement in pain over placebo without a significant increase in side effects. Oxycodone 20 mg controlled release tablets had greater efficacy, but adverse effects were also increased [13]. The American College of Rheumatology Subcommittee on Osteoarthritis Guidelines also agree that opioid therapy may be necessary and is appropriate to treat pain that has not responded to other analgesic agents [12].

More recent OA guidelines from the Osteoarthritis Research Society International (OARSI) make similar recommendations. They recommend the use of weak opioids and narcotic analgesics for the treatment of refractory pain in patients with knee or hip OA, where other agents have been ineffective or are contraindicated [14]. Stronger opioids should be reserved for severe pain in exceptional circumstances [14].

The American Medical Directors Association (AMDA) advocates the use of opioids for moderate-to-severe acute pain that is not relieved by, or is unlikely to respond to other categories of analgesics [15]. Specifically, they comment on the judicious utilization of opioids in comfort care for patients in the long-term care setting. These guidelines advise not using meperidine, propoxyphene, pentazocine, butorphanol, and other agonist–antagonist combinations [15].

When starting patients on opioids, the AMDA recommends establishing the amount needed using immediate-release medications [15]. Once the required dose has been established, the regimen should be converted to a long-acting agent in order to provide continuous pain relief and reduce adverse events [15].

The American Geriatrics Society has a similar position on the use of opioids in the treatment of persistent pain in older persons [16]. Specifically, they recommend that all older adults with moderate-to-severe pain, pain related to functional impairment, or diminished quality of life due to pain should be considered for opioid therapy [16]. Frequent or continuous pain should be treated with around the clock dosing, and breakthrough pain should be anticipated and treated with a short-acting agent as needed [16]. They caution against exceeding maximum dosing recommendations when using combination agents as part of the analgesic regimen [16]. They also strongly recommend assessing for adverse effects and for attainment of therapeutic goals [16].

Adverse Effects/Precautions

Common adverse effects of opioid analgesics (i.e., constipation, nausea, vomiting, sedation, and respiratory depression) are an extension of their pharmacologic effect. Because older adults are more likely to be affected by the acute and chronic toxicities of opioids; however, opioids should be started at conservative doses and titrated carefully. Vigano et al. compared age, pain intensity, and opioid dose in patients with advanced cancer and compared patients <65 years, 65–74 years, and ≥75 years [17]. When age was treated as a categoric variable, statistically significant differences were observed in the morphine equivalent daily dose, with older patients requiring a lower equianalgesic dose. Therefore, this reinforces the concept of starting older adults on low doses of opioids, and slowly titrating to effect, while minimizing adverse effects.

Constipation is the most common adverse effect associated with long-term opioid therapy [18]. Tolerance to constipation does not develop, and it occurs with such predictability that most patients will require a laxative regimen prophylactically upon starting opioid therapy. Opioids decrease propulsive peristaltic waves in both the small and large intestines, allowing desiccation of the feces [3]. One commonly used bowel protocol combines use of a stimulant laxative (senna) plus a stool softener (docusate), which addresses both causes of opioid-induced constipation [19]. These drugs are available in combination (Senokot-S or generic) or they may be administered separately, increasing dosage to effect. Should this be unsuccessful, consider adding additional laxatives such as milk of magnesia, lactulose, or sorbitol. Fiber should be discouraged because it can exacerbate the situation.

Oral naloxone (an opioid antagonist) has been tried for refractory opioid-induced constipation with some success, but it may cause systemic opioid withdrawal [20, 21]. Methylnaltrexone (also an opioid antagonist) was recently approved by the FDA for the treatment of opioid-induced constipation in patients with advanced illness, when response to laxative therapy has not been sufficient [22]. Results show reversal of opioid-induced constipation without a lessening of analgesia or induction of withdrawal symptoms, as methylnaltrexone does not cross the blood–brain barrier [23]. Laxation was achieved with methylnaltrexone in 48% of study participants within 4 h versus 15% with placebo [23]. Common side effects were gastrointestinal in nature including abdominal pain, flatulence, nausea, and diarrhea [23]. Dosing is subcutaneous and weight-based every other day as needed with no more than one dose per 24 h period [22]. Dose adjustment is recommended for patients with creatinine clearance <30 ml/min [22]. Methylnaltrexone is contraindicated in patients with known or suspected mechanical gastrointestinal obstruction [22].

Nausea and vomiting frequently occur with opioid therapy, with an incidence of 10–40% [1, 24]. Assessment of nausea and vomiting should be carefully conducted, as the pathogenesis of the complaint will dictate the preferred drug therapy. For example, a patient who complains of early satiety, bloating, or postprandial vomiting may have delayed gastric emptying, which would be best treated with metoclopramide. Patients who complain of nausea with position changes, or vertigo may suffer from vestibular dysfunction. In this case, a trial of meclizine would be warranted. Constipation may also cause nausea, and the treatment is obviously an effective bowel regimen.

Nausea associated with the initiation of opioid therapy generally subsides within a few days. One common treatment strategy is to put the patient on an antiemetic agent such as haloperidol or prochlorperazine around the clock for 48 h, then reduce to "as needed" dosing. If the nausea persists, it may be prudent to rotate to a different opioid.

Opioids frequently cause sedation and cognitive impairment with the initiation of opioid therapy or with dosage increases. Initial sedation may be due to sleep deprivation in part, due to poor pain control. Tolerance generally develops to the sedation, but if it does not, several strategies may be employed, such as [1]

- Discontinue any nonessential CNS depressant medications
- Evaluate the patient for concurrent causes (i.e., sepsis, brain metastasis)
- Reduce opioid dosage by 25%
- Add an adjunctive analgesic, allowing opioid dosage reduction
- Add a psychostimulant (i.e., methylphenidate 2.5 mg with breakfast and lunch; increase to 10 mg per day, then to 20 mg per day as needed)
- Treat concurrent confused, agitated behavior or hallucinations with an antipsychotic agent such as haloperidol
- Opioid rotation.

Respiratory depression is one of the most feared and dangerous adverse effects of opioid therapy, but it is uncommon if the opioid is dosed appropriately and titrated carefully. It is critical that the patient be monitored for other signs of CNS depression such as somnolence and mental clouding and bradypnoea [1]. If the patient is arousable, and steady-state concentrations of the opioid have been achieved, the opioid dose should be withheld and administered at a lower dose once the patient has improved. Naloxone should only be administered, if the patient is becoming increasingly obtunded, is unarousable, or has severe respiratory depression [1]. The naloxone dose should be titrated against the respiratory rate, taking care not to give an excessive dose, which will reverse analgesia.

Other recently discovered potential adverse effects include endocrinological abnormalities such as hypogonadism and erectile dysfunction [6, 25]. Use of opioids in women has been associated with amenorrhea and decreased sex hormone levels [25]. Patients should be tested for hormonal deficiencies, if they report symptoms consistent with such deficiencies, such as decreased libido or sexual dysfunction [6]. Insufficient evidence exists, however, to recommend routine screening [6]. Opioid treatment may also be associated with neuropsychological changes such as decreased reaction times, psychomotor speed, and working memory [25].

Patients, families, caregivers, and practitioners frequently confuse the concepts of "physical dependence" and "addiction." Physical dependence, as defined by the American Pain Society, American Academy of Pain Medicine, and the American Society of Addiction Medicine, is "a state of adaptation that is manifested by a drug class specific withdrawal syndrome that can be produced by abrupt cessation, rapid dose reduction, decreasing blood level of the drug, and/or administration of an antagonist" [26]. Many medications may cause physical dependence, including opioids, benzodiazepines, corticosteroids, and a variety of cardiac medications. Should it become necessary to discontinue the medication, however, the practitioner would titrate down the dosage to avoid the withdrawal syndrome.

Addiction is defined as "a primary, chronic, neurobiologic disease, with genetic, psychosocial, and environmental factors influencing its development and manifestations. It is characterized by behaviors that include one or more of the following: impaired control over drug use, compulsive use, continued use despite harm, and craving" [16, 26]. Factors associated with drug abuse in older adults include female gender, social isolation, history of substance abuse, and history of mental illness [27]. The development of addiction is extremely rare in a population with no previous history of substance abuse or psychiatric illness [1, 16]. Some clinicians may also argue that underuse of opioids in the older adult population constitutes a larger problem [16]. The worry of addiction should not prevent a practitioner from ordering opioid therapy for an older adult, if the patient has not shown previous signs of drug abuse or diversion. For patients who do have a history of substance abuse or diversion, there are specific strategies that should be utilized to still allow pain management involving the use of opioids.

Even though the older adult is at a much lower risk of addiction and opioid misuse, prescription opioid diversion and misuse in general has placed an increasing burden on the health-care system and society, costing an estimated $9.5 billion in the USA in 2005 [16]. The Food and Drug Administration Amendments Act of 2007 (FDAAA) granted the FDA the authority to require submission and implementation of Risk Mitigation and Evaluation Strategies (REMS), in an effort to ensure that the drug's benefits outweigh its risks [28]. REMS components can include any of the following: medication guides; patient package inserts; a communication plan for health care providers; elements to ensure safe use including requirements for those who prescribe, dispense, or use the drug; and a timetable for REMS submission [28]. At the current time, there is no proposed standardization of REMS programs for different agents. The FDA may require the development of REMS prior to drug approval to ensure safety or postapproval, if the FDA becomes aware of new safety information and determines REMS are necessary to ensure that benefits continue to outweigh risks [29]. Additionally, the FDA emphasizes that collaboration will be necessary in order to find a balance between reducing misuse/abuse and maintaining access for patients [29].

Commonly Used Opioids

Morphine is considered to be the standard opioid against which all others are compared. Morphine may be administered by the parenteral route of administration (IM, SC, IV, epidural, and intrathecal), oral, or rectal. It is very hydrophilic and has a half life of about 2 h in patients with normal renal function. The duration of action of immediate-release morphine is approximately 4 h. There are several oral long-acting formulations of morphine (MS Contin, Oramorph SR, EndoMorph, Kadian, and Avinza) that are dosed every 12–24 h. Kadian and Avinza are capsules containing sustained-release morphine beads, which may be sprinkled on soft food such as applesauce. Embeda (extended release morphine sulfate and sequestered naltrexone hydrochloride) is an abuse-deterrent formulation recently approved for the management of moderate-to-severe pain when a continuous, around-the-clock opioid analgesic is needed for an extended period of time [30]. The morphine component provides effective pain relief, while the sequestered naltrexone core passes through the body with no effect when taken as directed. Embeda should not be crushed or chewed, as this will release the sequestered naltrexone core and can precipitate withdrawal in opioid-tolerant patients [30]. This is the first abuse-deterrent formulation to be approved by the FDA and multiple agents are in the pipeline and should come to market in the near future. Embeda is dosed once or twice daily and may alternatively be sprinkled on applesauce. Similar precautions in dosing should be followed as would be recommended for morphine. Pharmacokinetics have not been studied in older adults, so prudence with initial dosing and titration is recommended [30]. A study looking at the efficacy of Embeda in patients with moderate-to-severe pain due to osteoarthritis of the hip or knee found that Embeda resulted in significantly superior pain relief compared to placebo [30].

Morphine is metabolized by the liver, undergoing glucuronic conjugation, H-demethylation, hydrolysis, and oxidation. The primary metabolite is morphine-6-glucuronide, which may accumulate in patients with renal insufficiency, causing central nervous system excitation and myoclonus, nausea, and increased sedation [1, 31]. Older adults may have reduced renal function and may be at increased risk for metabolite accumulation.

Oxycodone is a synthetic morphine congener. It is also a short-acting opioid, dosed every 4 h. It is available in combination with acetaminophen (i.e., Percocet and Tylox) or aspirin (Percodan). It is available as a monotherapeutic analgesic in both immediate-release and sustained-release (OxyContin) oral preparations. The sustained-release tablet is dosed every 12 h. Oxycodone is metabolized to largely inactive metabolites; therefore, it may be a safer alternative in older adults with renal impairment. Limited data suggest that oxycodone is less likely to cause hallucinations than morphine [32]. It should be noted that when combined with nonopioids, e.g., acetaminophen, the nonopioid component will limit the amount of opioid that can be administered due to the ceiling for safety of the nonopioid medication.

Hydromorphone is a short-acting hydrogenated ketone of morphine. It may be administered by the oral, rectal, parenteral, and intraspinal routes. Hydromorphone is particularly useful when administered via continuous subcutaneous infusion as it is five to eight times more potent on a milligram per milligram basis compared with morphine, thus allowing equianalgesia with far less volume. Hydromorphone is metabolized to largely inactive metabolites, making it a possibly safer opioid in older adults with renal impairment. Oral hydromorphone is dosed every 3–4 h. A long-acting formulation was approved in 2004 under the tradename, palladone, indicated for the management of moderate-to-severe pain in opioid-tolerant patients requiring around the clock analgesia for an extended period of time [33]. Subsequently, in July 2005, it was voluntarily recalled from the market due to data showing that when taken concomitantly with alcohol, there may be a rapid increase in release of drug and corresponding levels of hydromorphone within the body, possibly leading to fatalities [34]. A new once-daily extended release formulation is currently being investigated using the OROS technology. OROS is an osmotic-controlled release oral delivery of medications and has not been associated with dose-dumping when coadministered with alcohol [35]. In phase 3 clinical trials, OROS hydromorphone has been shown to provide effective analgesia for up to 24 h compared to placebo [35]. A new drug application has been submitted to the FDA for approval.

Fentanyl is a semisynthetic opioid that is approximately 80–100 times more potent (on an mg per mg basis) than morphine [5]. A highly lipophilic opioid, fentanyl has a short half-life after bolus administration, but the elimination half-life is affected by the extent of fat sequestration [1]. Fentanyl may be administered by the parenteral, transdermal, or transmucosal routes of administration.

A transdermal formulation of fentanyl (duragesic and generics), indicated for the management of chronic pain, is available in five strengths (12, 25, 50, 75, and 100 mcg). The transdermal fentanyl product is not indicated for acute or postoperative pain, sporadic pain, or patients who are not tolerant to opioid therapy due to the risk of serious or life-threatening hypoventilation [36]. Patients considered opioid tolerant are those who are taking at least 60 mg morphine/day, 25 mcg transdermal fentanyl/h, 30 mg of oxycodone daily 8 mg oral hydromorphone daily, or an equi-analgesic dose of another opioid for a week or longer [37]. This system is applied to the skin surface and changed every 3 days. After the patch is applied to the skin, serum concentrations increase, achieving serum concentrations required to produce analgesia by 12–16 h, and taking 17–48 h to achieve steady state [36]. The elimination half-life after transdermal patch removal ranges from 13 to –25 h; however, in older adults the elimination half-life more closely approximates 43.1 h [36]. Holdsworth et al. compared transdermal fentanyl disposition in elderly subjects to that in younger patients [38]. Application of a 20-cm² fentanyl 24-h transdermal patch (designed to deliver 40 μg/h) was compared in patients aged 67–87 years vs. those aged 19–27 years. All ten elderly subjects required patch removal prior to 24 h due to the development of side effects (notably nausea, vomiting, and respiratory distress) and had a significantly higher mean area under the curve from 0 to 60 h. The package insert for this product states, "Since elderly, cachectic, or debilitated patients may have altered pharmacokinetics due to poor fat stores, muscle wasting, or altered clearance, they should not be started on Duragesic doses higher than 25 μg/h unless they are already taking more than 135 mg of oral morphine a day or an equivalent dose of another opioid" [37]. Patients should be carefully titrated on trandermal fentanyl as many variables affect the delivery of fentanyl from the patch, including heat-associated increase in absorption [39, 40, 41].

Fentanyl is also available in three short-acting, transmucosal formulations. It is available as a buccal tablet (Fentora), a buccal lozenge (Actiq), and most recently a buccal soluble film (Onsolis). All three agents are indicated for breakthrough pain in chronic cancer patients already tolerant to opioid therapy. Each agent has a unique pharmacokinetic profile displaying differing bioavailability. The soluble film is 71% bioavailable compared to the lozenge and the tablet, which are only 47 and 65% bioavailable, respectively [42]. Substitution of the lozenge or the tablet with the film could, therefore, result in a significant overdose [42, 43]. Dosing strategies are dissimilar among the three rapid-acting fentanyl products, and conversion between these products is not recommended. The safety profile of Actiq and Onsolis in older adults did not differ from that of the younger cohort, but caution is advised in the individual titration of these products due to potential for increased sensitivity of this population to fentanyl products [42]. It is recommended that Fentora is dosed with caution as well in the older adult as there was a slight increase in adverse effects and a slightly lower dose was required in this population [43]. Of note, dispensing of the buccal film is done through the FOCUS program, developed as part of the FDA Risk Evaluation and Mitigation Strategy (REMS) initiative [42].

Oxymorphone is a synthetic opioid with higher potency than morphine or oxycodone, and a more rapid onset. It is available in both an immediate-release (Opana) and extended-release formulations (Opana ER). Studies in low back pain and osteoarthritis of the hip and knee demonstrated efficacy and safety in older adults with a mean age between 50 and 60 [44]. Levels of oxymorphone ER were found to be 40% higher in older adults compared with younger subjects and therefore slow titration is imperative in the older adult [44]. Oxymorphone should be used with caution in patients who are sensitive to CNS depressants and those with significant cardiovascular, pulmonary, renal, or hepatic disease [44]. Oxymorphone does not display significant drug interactions with the cytochrome P450 system [44].

Tramadol is an aminocyclohexanole derivative with weak opioid agonist activity. The drug has slight preference for the μ-opioid receptor, with an affinity approximately 6,000-fold less than that of morphine [45]. Tramadol also inhibits norepinephrine and serotonin reuptake [45]. Tramadol is indicated for the management of moderate-to-moderately severe pain. Tramadol may be used when patients wish to avoid or cannot tolerate opioids, but nonopioids are insufficient to manage pain, and may be used in combination with acetaminophen or an NSAID agent. Tramadol may also be used when acetaminophen is insufficient, but the patient is unable to tolerate the NSAID. The efficacy of tramadol is similar to that of equianalgesic doses of codeine and hydrocodone [46].

Tramadol has demonstrated efficacy in relieving painful conditions commonly experienced by older adults including osteoarthritis pain, chronic low back pain, painful diabetic neuropathy, and fibromyalgia pain [47]. Tramadol is also available in combination with acetaminophen (Ultracet®). This combination product is indicated for the short-term (5 days or less) management of acute pain. Each tablet contains 37.5 mg of tramadol, which is less than the monotherapeutic agent (50 mg per tablet) and 325 mg of acetaminophen. Prescribers should be careful to limit total daily acetaminophen dosage to 4,000 mg per day when using this combination analgesic, a limit that may be reduced in the near future. The combination may be particularly useful for older adults, as less tramadol is administered per tablet, thereby reducing the likelihood of adverse effects. Tramadol is also available as a once daily tablet formation (100, 200, and 300 mg).

Tramadol is not a controlled substance, and generally has low abuse potential in people without a previous history of substance abuse (not recommended in this population) [48].

The most common adverse effects of tramadol include dizziness, sedation, seizures, nausea, vomiting, and constipation [49]. Ruoff demonstrated that a slow initial titration of tramadol improves tolerability and reduces the discontinuation rate due to nausea, vomiting, dizziness, or vertigo [50]. Seizures have been reported with tramadol therapy [51]. Risk factors for seizures include dosages above the recommended range, concurrent therapy with certain medications (e.g., TCAs, selective serotonin reuptake inhibitors, opioids), or in patients with a history of seizures [47].

Short-acting tramadol can be administered as needed for relief every 4–6 h, not to exceed 400 mg per day. For patients over 75 years, not more than 300 mg/day in divided doses is recommended. The tramadol/acetaminophen combination (Ultracet) is administered in doses of two tablets every 4–6 h up to a maximum daily dosage of eight tablets. Tramadol requires dose adjustment in renal insufficiency and liver disease. The combination product requires renal dose adjustment and should be avoided in patient with hepatic disease due to the acetaminophen component.

The AMDA suggests that tramadol may be added to acetaminophen or an NSAID, or administered as monotherapy to manage chronic pain in the long-term care setting when patients have moderate-to-severe pain [15]. The American Pain Society and the American College of Rheumatology have suggested similar placement of tramadol in the treatment of osteoarthritis pain [12]. In the treatment of neuropathic pain, the IASP considers tramadol for use as a second-line agent or in combination with a first-line agent, as it is associated with significant side effects, a significant risk for misuse and abuse and has been shown to be less efficacious than first-line recommendations [11].

Tapentadol (Nucynta), a recently approved mu-opioid agonist and selective nor-epinephrine reuptake inhibitor, is similar in structure and mechanism of action to tramadol. Unlike tramadol, tapentadol is a class II controlled drug substance and is only approved for use in moderate-to-severe acute pain. As a part of the REMS program, the FDA requires a medication guide with its dispensing. It has an intermediate potency, estimated to be two to three times lower than that of morphine [52]. Tapentadol is dosed every 4–6 h up to 600 mg daily without regard to meals. Maximum concentrations do not seem to be altered in older adults and subsequent dose adjustments are not necessary [53]. Tapentadol should be dose reduced in moderate liver impairment and is not recommended in severe renal or hepatic disease [53]. Given its noradrenergic mechanism of action, tapentadol should not be used within 14 days of the administration of a monoamine oxidase inhibitor as it may lower the seizure threshold, and caution should be exercised against the use of other serotonergic medications [53]. Other main adverse effects are similar to that of opioid medications, but studies suggest that it may be associated with less nausea and vomiting than oxycodone [54]. In phase 3 clinical trials, tapentadol was found noninferior to oxycodone 15 mg in postbunionectomy patients and was associated with less study withdrawals due to adverse effects [55]. Findings were similar in late-stage osteoarthritis patients, with tapentadol demonstrating noninferiority to oxycodone 10 mg, less withdrawals due to adverse effects, and significantly less gastrointestinal side effects [54].

Less Preferred Opioids

Codeine is a semisynthetic derivative of morphine, used to treat mild-to-moderate pain. Codeine is commonly administered in combination with acetaminophen or aspirin. Approximately 10% of the codeine dose is metabolized to morphine (the active drug moiety). Some patients lack the cytochrome p450 isoenzyme 2D6 that is required for the activation of codeine to morphine [5]. Codeine causes significant nausea, to such an extent that many patients claim "codeine allergy."

Meperidine is a synthetic opioid, with an active metabolite (normeperidine). Normeperidine may accumulate in older patients with decreased renal function and cause significant side effects including delirium and seizures [56]. Meperidine should not be used to treat pain in older adults and is not a preferred opioid for use in patients of any age.

Propoxyphene has been removed from the U.S. market. Propoxyphene has approximately one-half to one-third the potency of codeine, which is less than two 325 mg aspirin tablets and has been clinically equated to the efficacy of 650 mg of acetaminophen alone [57]. The Cochrane database gave propoxyphene with acetaminophen a level 1 evidence of low analgesia [57]. More importantly, propoxyphene is metabolized to norpropoxyphene, which accumulates with chronic dosing, especially in older adults. This active metabolite causes sedation and dizziness, increasing the fall risk in older adults. Norpropoxyphene can also produce pulmonary edema and cardiotoxicity, apnea, cardiac arrest, and death [58]. The FDA recently considered removing propoxyphene from the market in the USA on the advice of a FDA Advisory Committee, but decided instead to require increased warning about the risk of overdose in the package labeling [59]. The side effects, adverse effects, and drug interactions of this agent far outweigh any benefit, it may confer in the management of pain [57]. The American Geriatrics Society Guidelines for the Management of Persistent Pain in Older Adults do not recommend propoxyphene as a preferred agent in older adults [16].

Methadone is a synthetic opioid used to treat pain and opioid abstinence syndromes and heroin users [5]. Methadone is relatively inexpensive when compared with other opioids and may be a preferred opioid in the management of neuropathic pain due to antagonism of the NMDA (N-methyl-D-aspartate) receptor [60]. Methadone is a lipophilic drug with a long and variable half-life (10–75 h), tending to be longer in older patients [61]. Methadone may be used as a first-line analgesic, but is more commonly used as an alternate during opioid rotation. The difficulty comes in establishing the relative potency of methadone to morphine (or other opioids), because the dose ratio of methadone to morphine is inversely proportional to the daily morphine dose administered [62]. For example, the morphine/methadone dose ratio may be 2.5:1 at lower doses of morphine (<100 mg per day), and 14:1 or higher with higher daily doses of morphine (i.e., >300 mg per day) [62].

Methadone has also been associated with the development of Torsade de Pointes with very high dose methadone, particularly in patients with additional risk factors for the development of arrhythmias [63].

Methadone is growing in use due to the low cost. However, given the long and variable half-life, the attention to detail required when converting from other opioids to methadone, and the risk of arrhythmias with high dosages, methadone is probably not a first-line opioid in treating pain in older adults. In patients with a true morphine allergy, however, methadone is one potential treatment option. It should also be noted that the American Geriatrics Society's recently updated guidelines on the management of persistent pain in older persons recommend that methadone is not used as a first-line agent [16]. Both the AGS Guidelines and the Clinical Guidelines for the Use of Chronic Opioid therapy in Chronic Noncancer Pain recommend that only clinicians well versed in the use and risks of methadone should initiate it and titrate it cautiously [6, 16].

Summary

Opioids are indicated for the management of moderate-to-severe pain in older adults; however, care is required in initial agent selection, dosage selection, and titration. Morphine is the standard of comparison with opioids; however, older adults may be at risk for toxicity due to the activity of the morphine-6-glucuronide metabolite. Patients who require opioid therapy for chronic pain should receive a long-acting opioid (such as morphine, oxycodone, oxymorphone, or fentanyl). The use of an immediate-release opioid formulation for the management of breakthrough pain is at the discretion of the prescriber.

Opioids that should be avoided in older adults include propoxyphene, codeine, and meperidine. Methadone should be reserved for cases where careful attention can be paid to dosing; however, the long and variable half-life in older adults may effectively limit its utility.

The future of opioid prescribing will likely be greatly affected by the development of abuse-deterrent formulations and implementation of the REMS programs. As programs role out, it is left to be determined how this will affect patient access to adequate and timely pain management.

Adjuvant Analgesics

In cases where "traditional" analgesics (i.e., acetaminophen, NSAIDs, and opioids) do not completely alleviate pain, adjuvant drug therapy may be useful. These agents may enhance the effect or allow dosage reduction of commonly used analgesics, treat concurrent symptoms that exacerbate pain, or be more effective therapeutic agents in the treatment of specific pain syndromes. It is important for the practitioner to understand the role of adjuvant analgesics, including preferred drug selection in older adults.

NSAID agents have long been used to treat a wide spectrum of mild-to-moderate pain syndromes. NSAIDs may also serve as adjunctive therapy to treat specific pain complaints such as bone metastasis, soft-tissue infiltration, arthritis, serositis, and surgical pain [19]. NSAIDs have also been shown to allow opioid dosage reduction when administered concurrently. Refer to the previous chapter for a further discussion of NSAID agents in older adults.

Bisphosphonates (i.e., pamidronate disodium, zoledronic acid, and alendronate sodium) have been studied in patients with painful bone metastases [64]. It remains unclear, if the efficacy of bisphosphonates varies between tumor types or between the presence of different types of bone lesions [64]. Data are promising, however, for both pamidronate and clodronate [16, 64]. The main adverse events associated with bisphosphonate therapy are acute-phase reactions, GI adverse effects (i.e., nausea, vomiting, diarrhea, constipation, and esophagitis), renal toxicity, hypocalcemia, and osteonecrosis of the jaw [16, 64].

Pharmacologic properties of corticosteroids include the ability to reduce inflammation, edema, and neuronal excitability, to increase appetite, and reduce nausea [65]. Corticosteroids may be useful to treat pain due to acute nerve compression and headache, visceral distension, increased intracranial pressure, soft-tissue infiltration, bone pain, and neuropathic pain [19, 65]. Dexamethasone is frequently used as an adjunctive agent; however, betamethasone and methylprednisolone have also been used with success. As useful as corticosteroids are, their adverse effect profile is considerable and may worsen concomitant diseases experienced by the elderly. Toxicities seen early in therapy include hypertension, hyperglycemia, immunosuppression, gastrointestinal ulceration, and psychiatric disorders [65]. With long-term administration, adverse effects include Cushing's disease, osteoporosis, proximal myopathy, and aseptic necrosis of the bone [65]. If the patient has a life-limiting illness, it is important to frequently reevaluate the risk:benefit ratio of continuing corticosteroid therapy. The AGS guidelines for persistent pain in older adults recommend to maximize safety with low-dose, short-term administration or to use in patients near the end of life [16].

Neuropathic pain is frequently not completely controlled by opioids alone; however, the addition of an adjunctive agent may be very useful. Antidepressants (particularly TCAs such as amitriptyline, nortriptyline, and desipramine or selective serotonin–norepinephrine reuptake inhibitors such as duloxetine, venlafaxine, or milnacipran), calcium-channel $\alpha2\delta$-subunit ligands (gabapentin and pregabalin), first and second generation antiepileptics (i.e., carbamazepine, phenytoin, valproic acid, lamotrigine, oxcarbazepine, and topiramate), anesthetics and antiarrhythmic agents (i.e., lidocaine and mexiletine), and other agents (i.e., baclofen, corticosteroids, calcitonin, bisphosphonates, and capsaicin) have reports of benefits for neuropathic pain [66].

TCAs have long been considered a primary intervention for the treatment of many neuropathic pain syndromes. The International Association for the Study of Pain (IASP) recognizes TCAs, specifically desipramine and nortriptyline, as a first-line therapy in the treatment of neuropathic pain [11]. Clinical trials have demonstrated the efficacy of TCAs in treating painful diabetic neuropathy, PHN, central poststroke pain, and cancer-related neuropathic pain syndromes [66]. These agents probably act by inhibiting nociceptive pain pathways by blocking the reuptake of serotonin and norepinephrine. It is important to note that the selective serotonin reuptake inhibitor antidepressants (i.e., fluoxetine, paroxetine, and sertraline) have not demonstrated significant efficacy in treating neuropathic pain [67, 25, 10].

The adverse effects caused by TCAs are well recognized and include those related to their anticholinergic activity (constipation, dry mouth, blurred vision, urinary retention, cognitive changes, and tachycardia). Additional adverse effects include orthostatic hypotension, sedation, falls, weight gain, and potential lethality in overdose. Often, the adverse effect profile of this class of drugs contraindicates their use in older adults [16]. Generally speaking, the secondary amines (desipramine and nortriptyline) are preferred for older adults because they cause less anticholinergic and sedative effects than do the tertiary amines (i.e., amitriptyline) [66]. The AGS specifically recommends against the utilization of tertiary amine TCAs such as amitriptyline, imipramine, and doxepine in older adults [16]. TCAs should be administered cautiously to patients with preexisting conditions that could be worsened by the effects of these agents, including angle-closure glaucoma, benign prostatic hypertrophy, constipation, cardiovascular disease, or impaired liver function [66]. The dosage should be started low in older adults, such as 10 mg at bedtime (to minimize impact of sedation) and titrated up every 3–5 days as tolerated. A therapeutic effect should be seen in 3–10 days (more quickly than the antidepressant effect), generally at doses less than 100 mg per day. If one TCA does not adequately treat the neuropathic pain, it is worth a trial with a different agent (taper off the first agent).

The selective norepinephrine–serotonin reuptake inhibitors (SNRIs) are not associated with the anticholinergic side effects like those of the TCAs and may be better tolerated by the older adult. The IASP also considers this class of agents as a first-line option in the treatment of neuropathic pain [11]. Duloxetine (Cymbalta) is an SNRI that is indicated for the treatment of pain due to diabetic neuropathy or fibromyalgia. Duloxetine was proven superior to placebo in three 12-week trials in patients with painful diabetic neuropathy as well as a single 6-month trial in the treatment of fibromyalgia [25]. Recommended dosing for duloxetine in the treatment of neuropathic pain and fibromyalgia is 60 mg once daily and dosing greater than this was not found to be associated with greater efficacy [11]. Dose adjustments are necessary in renal dysfunction and caution should be used in patients with hepatic insufficiency. Because of reports of urinary retention, caution in men with prostatic hypertrophy should be exercised. Otherwise, duloxetine has a generally favorable side effect profile, most commonly associated with nausea that is best tolerated when therapy is slowly titrated from 30 to 60 mg over 1 week [11].

Venlafaxine (Effexor) is another SNRI that inhibits serotonin reuptake at lower doses and both serotonin and norepinephrine reuptake at higher doses [11]. Venlafaxine is available in a long-acting and an immediate-release formulation. Venlafaxine was found to be superior to placebo in a 6-week trial of patients with diabetic neuropathy at dosages between 150 and 225 mg/day and may be helpful in this condition, although it is not currently indicated for this use by the FDA [11, 25]. For maximum tolerability, venlafaxine should be slowly tapered to maximum effective dosage over 2–4 weeks and slowly tapered off upon discontinuation to avoid the discontinuation syndrome [11].

Milnacipran (Savella) is the newest addition to this class of agents and is indicated for the treatment of pain due to fibromyalgia. Milnacipran has been shown to result in significant improvement in pain and other symptoms of fibromyalgia after just 1 week of treatment [68]. Milnacipran should be tapered slowly to the effective dose with a maximum of 100 mg twice daily [69]. Dosing should be adjusted for severe renal impairment and use is not recommended in end-stage renal disease [69]. Treatment is most commonly associated with gastrointestinal symptoms, specifically nausea and constipation [68]. Elevations in blood pressure are also common and should be monitored for during treatment [69].

The antiarrythmic agent, lidocaine, is thought to work on voltage-gated sodium channels in peripheral nerves that are implicated in abnormally high rates of spontaneous firing. Lidocaine (2.5%) has been shown to be effective in reducing chronic neuropathic pain when applied in a cream in combination with 2.5% prilocaine (EMLA). Lidocaine, for the treatment of neuropathic pain, has been most frequently used in a topical patch formulation [44]. The patch provides peripheral analgesia as well as a mechanical barrier that reduces allodynia. Topical lidocaine 5% patches (Lidoderm) are considered a first-line therapy in the treatment of neuropathic pain by the IASP [11]. While only indicated for the treatment of PHN, lidocaine 5% patches have also been shown to be effective in patients with diverse peripheral neuropathic conditions and allodynia [11]. The American Geriatrics Society also recognizes the role of the lidocaine 5% patch in the treatment of PHN but states that the benefit does not compare with that of gabapentin or TCAs [16].

The only side effects associated with the use of the lidocaine 5% patch are local skin reactions. Given such a safe adverse event profile and minimal potential for drug interactions, the lidocaine patch is a good option for the older adult with local peripheral neuropathies [44]. Suggested dosing for the lidocaine patch is up to three patches on for 12 h and then off for 12 h. Of note, 95% of the medication remains in the patch after 12 h of application [44]. Blood levels for four patches applied for up to 24 h are still minimal with plasma levels at 12–15% of the lidocaine levels required for cardiac activity and 4–5% of those that cause toxicity [44]. Despite minimal systemic absorption, the lidocaine patch should not be used in patients on oral Class I antiarrhythmic medications or in patients with severe hepatic dysfunction due to decreased clearance Lidocaine gel has demonstrated efficacy in HIV neuropathy and can be considered in place of the patch if it is unavailable, application is a problem or the cost of the patch is an issue [11].

Gabapentin (Neurontin) and pregabalin (Lyrica) are very popular and have strong evidence in the treatment of neuropathic pain. They most likely act via the $\alpha2\delta$-subunit protein of calcium channels in regions of the brain and the superficial horn of the spinal cord causing a decrease in excitatory neurotransmitters involved in the transmission of the pain signal [11, 25]. The tolerability and efficacy of the gabapentinoids, treating a variety of pains including reflex sympathetic dystrophy, diabetic neuropathy, trigeminal neuropathy, PHN, radiation myelopathy, central poststroke pain, neuropathic cancer pain, and fibromyalgia have contributed to their popularity [66]. Gabapentin and pregabalin have been recommended as first-line anticonvulsants in the treatment of neuropathic pain [11, 25]. In addition to being efficacious, gabapentin and pregabalin have fewer adverse effects and drug interactions than most other neuropathic pain therapies. The major adverse effects associated with gabapentinoids are sedation, dizziness, ataxia, and fatigue [70]. Tolerance generally develops to these adverse effects; however, it is prudent to begin therapy at a low dose, and titrate to effect. Dosing for gabapentin generally begins at 100 mg three times daily, although some older adults may be better served by starting with 100 mg once or twice daily to start. Titrate to effect, balancing against side effects. Most patients who respond will usually do so at total daily doses of 900–1,800 mg. Some practitioners have pushed the daily dosage higher, if a partial response is seen by 1,800 mg per day. Although gabapentin is available as a generic medication, pregabalin has in its favor an easier dosing schedule (twice daily) and a possibly simpler dose titration.

Anticonvulsant agents are also considered relatively effective treatments of a wide variety of neuropathic pain complaints, particularly with lancinating, or tic-like pain. The IASP places these agents in the category of third-line options due to substantially less evidence supporting their efficacy as agents such as the TCAs, SNRIs, and calcium channel $\alpha2\delta$ ligands [11].

The first generation anticonvulsants such as carbamazepine, phenytoin, and valproic acid, and the second generation anticonvulsants such as oxcarbazepine, lamotrogine and topiramate, probably act by increasing membrane stability (as seen with seizures). Clonazepam has also been used to treat neuropathic pain, and it acts by enhancing γ-aminobutyric acid $(GABA)_A$-receptor-mediated inhibition. The AGS recommends against the use of benzodiazepines as evidence of efficacy is limited and there is a high risk of cognitive changes in older adults [16].

Carbamazepine has been used to treat painful diabetic neuropathy and trigeminal neuralgia [71]. Carbamazepine autoinduces its own hepatic metabolism, which requires the practitioner start at low doses (i.e., 100 mg po twice daily) and increase the dosage weekly to the therapeutic dose (approximately 1,200 mg po qd, although dosages up to 1,600 mg/day have been necessary pain relief) [66]. Carbamazepine is responsible for many drug interactions due to its ability to induce hepatic enzyme activity. Adverse effects include CNS effects (drowsiness, vertigo, ataxia, diplopia, and blurred vision), gastrointestinal effects (nausea and vomiting), serious hematologic toxicity (aplastic anemia and agranulocytosis), transient increase in hepatic enzymes, and hypersensitivity reactions (dermatitis, eosinophilia, lymphadenopathy, and splenomegaly) [72].

Phenytoin has also been used to treat a variety of neuropathic pain complaints. Careful attention to detail is required with phenytoin dosing, because the drug exhibits "capacity-limited," or "storability" metabolism. At therapeutic concentrations, the rate of metabolism is close to the limit, and small dosage increases may result in significantly higher serum concentrations. Phenytoin is also highly bound to serum albumin, and a higher "free" or "unbound" fraction would be expected in patients who are hypoalbuminemic, potentially causing toxicity despite a therapeutic "total" phenytoin serum concentration. Phenytoin is involved in many drug interactions with other medications that are also highly protein bound. Chronic phenytoin dosing and toxicity include adverse effects such as dose-related cerebellar-vestibular effects, CNS effects, behavioral changes, increased frequency of seizures, gastrointestinal symptoms, gingival hyperplasia, osteomalacia, and megaloblastic anemia. Older adults are at greater risk for phenytoin-related toxicity [72]. It is also worth mentioning that phenytoin can adversely diminish vitamin D status, a problem commonly seen in older patients [73].

Second generation anticonvulsants have been studied in several trials. Data on the efficacy of all three agents (lamotrogine, oxcarbazepine, and topiramate) are conflicting [11]. Of note, it is important to be mindful of the need to slowly titrate lamotrogine to reduce the risk of serious cutaneous hypersensitivity reactions.

Other medications that may be used to treat neuropathic pain adjunctively include mexiletine, clonidine, lidocaine, baclofen, corticosteroids, calcitonin, capsaicin, bisphosphonates (pamidronate), strontium chloride, ketamine, and dronabinol [19, 65, 66, 74, 75, 76].

Summary

Older adults suffer from many chronic conditions that are likely to have a painful component. It is imperative that practitioners develop excellent skills in detecting and assessing pain, selecting the most appropriate analgesic regimen, and monitoring for efficacy and potential toxicity.

References

1. Cherny CI. Opioid analgesics. Comparative features and prescribing guidelines. Drugs. 1996;51:713–37.
2. Matthew MT, Nance PW. Analgesics. Opioid, adjuvants and others. Phys Med Rehabil Clin N Am. 1999;10:255–73.
3. Butstein HB, Akil H. Opioid analgesics. In: Hardman JG, Limbird LE, editors. Goodman & Gilman's the pharmacological basis of therapeutics. 10th ed. New York: McGraw-Hill; 2001. p. 569–619.
4. Jacox AK, Carr DB, Payne R, Berde CB, Breitbart W, Cain JM, et al. Management of Cancer Pain Guideline No. 9. AHCPR Pub. No. 94–0592. Rockville, MD: Agency for Health Care Policy and Research, Publich Health Service, U.S. Department of Health and Human Services; 1994.
5. Staats P, Johnson R. New perspectives on the pharmacology of opioids and their use in chronic pain. A Dannemiller Pain Management Monograph. 2001. http://www.pain.com/articles/onepage.cfm?chapter_id=85. Accessed 4 Nov 2002.
6. Chou R, Fanciullo GJ, Fine PG, Adler JA, Ballantyne JC, Davies P, et al. Clinical guidelines for the use of chronic opioid therapy in chronic noncancer pain. J Pain. 2009;10(2):113–30. WHO 2009.
7. World Health Organization. WHO's pain ladder. http://www.who.int/cancer/palliative/painladder/en/ (2009). Accessed 10 Nov 2009.
8. Zech D, Grond S, Lynch J, Hertel D, Lehmann KA. Validation of World Health Organization Guidelines for cancer pain relief: a 10 year prospective study. Pain. 1989;17:1281.
9. Eisenberg E, Marinangeli F, Birkhahn J, Paladini A, Varrassi G. Time to modify the WHO analgesic ladder? IASP Pain: Clin Updates. 2005;XIII(5):1–4.
10. Mercadente S, Arcuri E. Pharmacological management of cancer pain in the elderly. Drugs Aging. 2007;24(9):761–76.
11. Dworkin RH, O'Connor AB, Backonja M, Farrar JT, Finnerup NB, Jensen TS, et al. Pharmacologic management of neuropathic pain: evidence-based recommendations. Pain. 2007;132:237–51.
12. American College of Rheumatology Subcommittee on Osteoarthritis Guidelines. Recommendations for the medical management of osteoarthritis of the hip and knee. Arthritis Rheum. 2002;43:1905–15.
13. Roth SH, Fleischmann RM, Burch FX, Dietz F, Bockow B, Rapoport RJ, et al. Around-the-clock, controlled-release oxycodone therapy for osteoarthritis-related pain: placebo-controlled trial and long-term evaluation. Arch Intern Med. 2000;160:853–60.
14. OARSI recommendations for the management of hip and knee osteoarthritis, Part II. OARSI evidence-based, expert consensus guidelines. Osteoarthr Cartil. 2008;16:137–62.
15. American Medical Directors Association. Chronic pain management in the long-term care setting. 2009.
16. AGS Panel on the Pharmacological Management of Persistent Pain in Older Persons. Pharmacological management of persistent pain in older persons. J Am Geriatr Soc. 2009;57:1331–46.
17. Vigano O, Bruera E, Suarez-Almazor ME. Age, pain intensity, and opioid dose in patients with advanced cancer. Cancer. 1998;83:1244–50.
18. Portenyo RK. Management of common opioid side effects during long-term therapy of cancer pain. Ann Acad Med Singapore. 1994;23(2):160–70.
19. Levy MH. Pharmacologic treatment of cancer pain. N Engl J Med. 1996;335:1124–32.
20. Sykes NP. Oral naloxone in opioid associated constipation. Lancet. 1991;337:1475.
21. Culpepper-Morgan JA, Inturrisi CE, Portenoy RK, Foley K, Houde RW, Marsh F, et al. Treatment of opioid induced constipation with oral naloxone: a pilot study. Clin Pharmacol Ther. 1992;52:90–95.
22. Relistor Package Insert. http://www.wyeth.com/content/showlabeling.asp?id=499 (2009). Accessed 13 Nov 2009.

23. Thomas J, Karver S, Cooney GA, Chamberlain BH, Watt CK, Slatkin NE, et al. Methylnaltrexone for opioid-induced constipation in advanced illness. N Engl J Med. 2008;358:2332–43.
24. Campora E, Merlini L, Pace M, et al. The incidence of narcotic induced emesis. J Pain Symptom Manage. 1991;6:428–30.
25. Kroenke K, Krebs EE, Bair MJ. Pharmacotherapy of chronic pain: a synthesis of recommendations from systematic reviews. Gen Hosp Psychiatry. 2009;31:206–19.
26. American Academy of Pain Medicine, American Pain Society and American Society of Addiction Medicine. Definitions related to the use of opioids for the treatment of pain. 2003. American Academy of Pain Medicine Web Page, http://www.painmed.org/productpub/statements/ (2003). Accessed 10 Mar 2003.
27. Culberson JW, Ziska M. Prescription drug misuse/abuse in the elderly. Geriatrics. 2008;63(9):22–6, 31.
28. FDA News Release. FDA issues draft guidance on risk evaluation and mitigation strategies. 2009. http://www.fda.gov/NewsEvents/Newsroom/PressAnnouncements/ucm184399.htm Accessed 21 Nov 2009.
29. Jenkins, John. REMS and opioid analgesics Webinar. FDA. 2009. http://www.fda.gov. Accessed 21 Nov 2009.
30. Embeda Package Insert. http://ww.embeda.com (2009). Accessed 17 Nov 2009.
31. Hagen NA, Foley KM, Cerbone DJ, Portenoy RK, Inturrisi CE. Chronic nausea and morphine-6-glucuronide. J Pain Symptom Manage. 1991;6:125–8.
32. Poyhia R, Vainio A, Kalso E. A review of oxycodone's clinical pharmacokinetics and pharmacodynamics. Curr Ther Res. 1978;24:633–45.
33. Thomson Healthcare Inc. Hydromorphone. Drugpoint summary. http://ww.thomsonhc.com. Accessed 23 Nov 2009.
34. Memorandum. Overview of the September 23, 2009 ALSDAC meeting to discuss NDA 21–217 for Exalgo, an extended–release formulation of hydromorphone. FDA Center for Drug Evaluation and Research; August 2009.
35. Weinstein SM. A new extended release formulation (OROS) of hydromorphone in the management of pain. Ther Clin Risk Manag. 2009;5:75–80.
36. Jeal W, Benfield P. Transdermal fentanyl: a review of its pharmacological properties and therapeutic efficacy in pain control. Drugs. 1997;53:109–38.
37. Duragesic package insert. http://www.duragesic.com/files/duragesic_pres_info.pdf (2009). Accessed 10 Nov 2009.
38. Holdsworth MT, Forman WB, Killilea TA, Nystrom KM, Paul R, Brand SC, et al. Transdermal fentanyl disposition in elderly subjects. Gerontology. 1994;40:32–7.
39. Marquardt KA, Tharratt RS, Musallam NA. Fentanyl remaining in a transdermal system following three days of continuous use. Ann Pharmacother. 1995;29:969–71.
40. Carter KA. Heat-associated increase in transdermal fentanyl absorption. Am J Health Syst Pharm. 2003;60:191–2.
41. Newshan G. Heat-related toxicity with the fentanyl transdermal patch. J Pain Symptom Manage. 1998;16:277–8.
42. Onsolis package insert. http://www.onsolis.com/pdf/onsolis_pi.pdf. Accessed 10 Nov 2009.
43. Fentora Package Insert. http://www.fentora.com/pdfs/pdf100_prescribing_info.pdf. Accessed 10 Nov 2009.
44. McGeeney BE. Pharmacological management of neuropathic pain in older adults: an update on peripherally and centrally acting agents. J Pain Symptom Manage. 2009;38: S15–27.
45. Radbruch L, Grond S, Lehmann KA. A risk-benefit assessment of tramadol in the management of pain. Drug Saf. 1996;15:8–29.
46. AGS Panel on Persistent Pain in Older Persons. The management of persistent pain in older persons. J Am Geriatr Soc. 2002;50:1–20.

47. Schnitzer TJ. Managing chronic pain with tramadol in elderly patients. Clin Geriatr. 1999;7(8):http://www.mmhc.com/cg/v7n8.shtml. Accessed 18 Feb 2003.
48. Cicero TJ, Adams EH, Geller A, Inciardi JA, Munoz A, Schnoll SH, et al. A postmarketing surveillance program to monitor Ultram (tramadol hydrochloride) abuse in the United States. Drug Alcohol Depend. 1999;57:7–22.
49. RxList Tramadol. www.rxlist.com/cgi/generic/tramadol_ids.htm. Accessed 11 Nov 2009.
50. Ruoff GE. Slowing the initial titrate rate of tramadol improves tolerability. Pharmacotherapy. 1999;19:88–93.
51. Kahn LH, Alderfer RJ, Graham DJ. Seizures reported with tramadol. JAMA. 1997;278:1661.
52. Tzschentke TM, Christoph T, Kogel B, Schien K, Hennies HH, Englberger W, et al. Tapentadol HCL: a novel u-opioid receptor agonist/norepinephrine reuptake inhibitor with broad-spectrum analgesic properties. J Pharmacol Exp Ther. 2007;323(1):265–76.
53. Tapentadol Package Insert. http://www.nucynta.com/nucynta/assets/Nucynta-PI.pdf. Accessed 17 Nov 2009.
54. Hartrick C, Van Hove I, Stegmann JU, Oh C, Upmalis D. Efficacy and tolerability of tapentadol immediate release and oxycodone HCl immediate release in patients awaiting primary joint replacement surgery for end-stage joint disease: a 10-day, phase III, randomized, double-blind, active- and placebo-controlled study. Clin Ther. 2009;31(2):260–71.
55. Daniels SE, Upmalis D, Okamoto A, Lange C, Haeussler J. A randomized, double-blind, phase III study comparing multiple doses of tapentadol IR, oxycodone IR, and placebo for postoperative (bunionectomy) pain. Curr Med Res Opin. 2009;25(3):765–76.
56. Clark RF, Wei EM, Anderson PO. Meperidine: therapeutic use and toxicity. J Emerg Med. 1995;13:797–802.
57. Barkin RL, Barkin SJ, Barkin DS. Propoxyphene (Dextropropoxyphene): a critical review of a weak opioid analgesic that should remain in antiquity. Am J Ther. 2006;13:534–42.
58. Perin ML. Problems with propoxyphene. Am J Nurs. 2000;100:22.
59. Food and Drug Administration. Propoxyphene questions and answers. http://www.fda.gov/Drugs/DrugSafety/PostmarketDrugSafetyInformationforPatientsandProviders/ucm170268.htm. Accessed 29 Nov 2009.
60. Cleary JF. Methadone: the ideal long-acting opioid? AAHPM Bulletin Winter. 2002;13:6–7.
61. Wheeler WL, Dickerson ED. Clinical applications of methadone. Am J Hosp Palliat Care. 2002;17:196–203.
62. Davis MP, Walsh D. Methadone for relief of cancer pain: a review of pharmacokinetics, pharmacodynamics, drug interactions and protocols of administration. Support Care Cancer. 2001;9:73–83.
63. Krantz MJ, Lawkowiez LL, Hays H, Woodroffe MA, Robertson AD, Mehler PS. Torsade de Pointes associated with very-high-dose methadone. Ann Intern Med. 2002;137:501–4.
64. Gralow J, Tripathy D. Managing metastatic bone pain: the role of bisphosphonates. J Pain Symptom Manage. 2007;33:462–72.
65. Goldstein FJ. Adjuncts to opioid therapy. J Am Osteopath Assoc. 102(9):S15–21.
66. Guay DRP. Adjunctive agents in the management of chronic pain. Pharmacotherapy. 2001;21:1070–81.
67. McQuay HJ, Tramer M, Nye BA, Carroll D, Wiffen PJ, Moore RA. A systematic review of antidepressants in neuropathic pain. Pain. 1996;68:217–27.
68. Clauw DJ, Mease P, Palmer RH, Gendreau RM, Wang Y. Milnacipran for the treatment of fibromyalgia in adults: a 15-week, multicenter, randomized, double-blind, placebo-controlled, multiple-dose clinical trial (abstract). Clin Ther. 2008;30(11):1988–2004.
69. Milnacipran Package Insert. http://www.frx.com/pi/Savella_pi.pdf. Accessed 22 Nov 2009.
70. Ross EL. The evolving role of antiepileptic drugs in treating neuropathic pain. Neurology. 2000;55(Suppl 1):S41–46.
72. Sindrup SH, Jensen TS. Efficacy of pharmacological treatments of neuropathic pain: an update and effect related to mechanism of drug action. Pain. 1999;83:389–400.

73. McNamara JO. Drugs effective in the therapy of the epilepsies. In: Hardman JG, Limbird LE, editors. Goodman and Gilman's the pharmacologic basis of therapeutics. 10th ed. New York: McGraw-Hill; 2001. p. 521–47.
74. Gloth III, FM, Tobin JDA. Review of Vitamin D deficiency in the elderly: what we know and what we don't. J Am Geriatr Soc. 1995;43:822–8.
75. Watson CPN. Topical capsaicin as an adjuvant analgesic. J Pain Symptom Manage. 1994;9:425–33.
76. Mao J, Chen LL. Systemic lidocaine for neuropathic pain relief. Pain. 2000;87:7–17.

Chapter 9
Interventional Strategies for Pain Management

Kulbir S. Walia, Frederick W. Luthardt, Maneesh C. Sharma,
and Peter S. Staats

> *Do not rashly use every new product of which the peripatetic*
> *siren sings.*
>
> Sir William Osler

The International Association for the Study of Pain (IASP) defines pain as "an unpleasant sensory and emotional experience associated with actual or potential tissue damage, or described in terms of such damage." While pain is traditionally thought of as a part of the body's defense system, triggering a reflex reaction to retract or withdraw from a painful stimulus, in certain circumstances, it becomes a disease in and of itself.

Usually acute pain stops without treatment or responds to simple measures such as resting or taking analgesic drugs, but sometimes pain becomes chronic and unresponsive to simpler measures. The geriatric population has a high incidence of diseases that can cause unremitting pain, including cancer, arthritis, and spinal disorders. In addition to the adverse effects on the quality of life from the disease itself, uncontrolled pain shortens one's life expectancy and decreases the quality of life [1].

A good general paradigm is to begin with conservative therapies to treat pain and gradually move up a spectrum of invasiveness. This usually involves beginning with systemic oral and transdermal medications [2]. But conservative therapies do not always relieve pain, and a significant minority of patients would benefit from interventional therapies. Furthermore, conservative therapies sometimes relieve pain only by substituting equally untenable side effects. These side effects, which can be triggered by pharmaceuticals or even by a seemingly innocuous therapy such as bed rest, are more likely to occur and to have a heightened impact in older adults.

P.S. Staats (✉)
Department of Anesthesiology and Critical Care Medicine, Department of Oncology at
Johns Hopkins, University School of Medicine in Baltimore, Maryland,
Premier Pain Management, Shrewsbury, NJ, USA
e-mail: pstaats@jhmi.edu

F.M. Gloth, III (ed.), *Handbook of Pain Relief in Older Adults: An Evidence-Based Approach*, Aging Medicine, DOI 10.1007/978-1-60761-618-4_9,
© Springer Science+Business Media, LLC 2011

When conservative therapies have failed or there are rate limiting side effects, clinicians should always consider using interventional pain management techniques. Interventional pain treatment should be offered to patients with terminal diseases in whom such aggressive therapy may appear, at first glance, to be counterintuitive [1, 3, 4]. They should also be offered to patients with long-life expectancy, who will benefit from the therapies for years to come.

Understanding the Pathology of the Pain

Over the past decades, pain practitioners have recognized that there has been an undertreatment of pain and encouraged opioid prescribing. The World Health Organization ladder has been lauded as a method for encouraging appropriate use of opioids in the management of pain. In this paradigm, if a patient has mild pain, nonsteroidals are used; for moderate pain, weak opioids are used; and with severe pain, strong opioids are used [5].

This paradigm does not question the pathology or consider other strategies. It is my view that this is too simplistic for modern day pain management. A thorough understanding of the pathophysiology and disease process would, on the other hand, lead to more specific therapies that may lead to improved pain relief and a lower side-effect profile [6]. They, in essence, can block the pain at its source, or modulate the transmission of pain. It is important to begin with a thorough history and physical examination in order to define the pathology, and thus develop the most appropriate treatment strategy. This can be supplemented with diagnostic studies that will facilitate an accurate diagnosis.

Identification of the origin of the pain will point to sympathetic, somatic, visceral, central, or even psychogenic mechanisms. After the mechanism is diagnosed, a treatment plan can be formulated and may include the use of interventional strategies to block pain transmission. This chapter will provide an introduction to many of the most common and some of the newest of these interventions and their effectiveness in treating pain.

Pathophysiology of Pain

In most cases, pain is transmitted from peripheral pain generators (nociceptors) to the spinal cord, where it proceeds up the lateral spinothalamic tract to the frontal cortex, which is responsible for the perception of pain. At every stage of transmission, pain can be modulated (see Fig. 9.1) [7]. Interventional therapies (1) affect pain generators (leaky disk, inflamed nerve, etc.) by blocking transmission of nociception, (2) enhance the body's own pain control system, using neuromodulation techniques (spinal cord stimulation), or (3) capitalize on local receptors or nerves or spinal cord (and, thus, use exceedingly low doses of

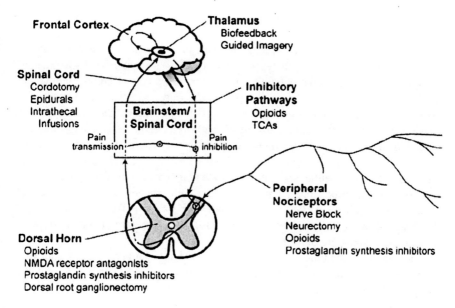

Fig. 9.1 Pain Transmission pathway and Modulation strategies

pharmacologic agents (intrathecal pumps). By minimizing nociception and pain transmission, analgesic doses of medications required to control pain can be minimized.

Nerve Blocks

Use of Local Anesthetics to Block a Nerve

Injection of a local anesthetic to achieve a temporary block in transmission of chronic non-cancer pain and pain generated by the sympathetic nervous system sometimes allows us to predict what will happen if we attempt to destroy a nerve. In addition to performing such diagnostic nerve blocks, we also treat a variety of painful conditions arising from cancer by blocking nerves with repeated injections or a continuous infusion of local anesthetics.

The procedure is simple: to block a nerve, we infuse the area around the nerve with a local anesthetic (often mixed with a steroid). Myoneural injections are performed in the location of trigger points, which are distinct localized areas of tenderness within a taut band of muscle running parallel to the direction of the muscle fibers. These tender areas are hard and are linear or nodular in shape. Palpation can cause pain, produce altered sensations, or elicit a local twitch response. Trigger points can be treated by inserting a dry needle into the site and, then, manipulating the needle to break up the congested area. Sometimes we also inject small amounts of a local anesthetic or of botulinum toxin into the target muscle.

Any intervention carries a risk inherent to the procedure itself. The risks and benefits of all procedures must, therefore, be weighed. With nerve blocks, one should always be cognizant of the patient's coagulation status and bleeding time. Certain malignancies and anticoagulation therapy can alter blood chemistry and increase the possibility of the procedure causing bleeding into the site or neuraxis, which can cause permanent nerve damage, paralysis, and even death. Other factors that may contraindicate nerve block injections are hypovolemia, dehydration, and cachexia.

As noted, local anesthetic nerve blocks are performed for three purposes: they are diagnostic, therapeutic, and can serve to help predict the results of more permanent or ablative procedures. Diagnostic nerve blocks are done to differentiate between the mechanisms that may be responsible for the patient's persistent pain. As there are many mechanisms that can cause pain, there are also many types of nerve blocks; some are described below.

Therapeutic nerve blocks are performed to alleviate pain complaints after diagnosis. Injection of a local anesthetic with or without a steroid can provide relief of symptoms. There is also evidence that a repeat series of injections may provide long-term pain relief.

Evidence about the efficacy of nerve blocks in general, however, is contradictory. A review of the published reports up to 1997 was inconclusive about the efficacy of epidural injections in low back pain and sciatica [8]. Koes et al. conducted a similar review in 1995 and drew a similar conclusion [9]. Other investigators, however, find epidural injections an effective treatment for sciatica [10]. Part of the problem may rest with variations in the method used to administer the injections or in degrees of proficiency in appropriate patient selection. Or, as suggested by Hopayian and Mugford, the origin of the discrepancy may simply lie in the difference in thechoice of methods used to conduct the systematic review [11].

Blocking Specific Sites

Facet Blocks

The small, diarthrodial facet joints provide posterior support to the spine. As people age, they can develop arthritis that is associated with severe pain in these joints. There are two types of blocks: intra-articular and posterior rami blocks. Facet blocks are performed in the lumbar, thoracic, or cervical spine. A patient with facet syndrome may experience tenderness in the area of the facet joints, pain upon movement or twisting of the spine, or local muscle spasms and/or hyperalgesia. Pain is generally exacerbated with ipsilateral extension of the spine. Discomfort on the contralateral side, however, is more consistent with myofascial pain.

Patients with lumbar facet syndrome experience a deep, dull ache unilaterally or bilaterally in the lower back, and this pain may radiate to the buttock, groin, or hip or from the posterior thigh to the knee. Patients with short-term low back pain, thought to be consistent with lumbar facet pain, can be considered for intra-articular steroids [12]. If pain persists, a denervation is indicated (see below).

ASIPP (American Society of Interventional Pain Physicians) Systematic Review [13] concludes that the accuracy of facet joint nerve blocks is strong in the diagnosis of lumbar facet joint pain. The evidence for short- and long-term improvement in managing low back pain with intra-articular injections of local anesthetics and steroids is moderate. The evidence is moderate for short- and long-term pain relief with lumbar medial branch blocks in managing chronic low back pain.

The evidence for radiofrequency neurotomy of medial branches in the cervical and lumbar regions is strong for short-term and moderate for long-term relief. The evidence for cryodenervation and pulsed radiofrequency is indeterminate.

Sacroiliac Joint Injections

The sacroiliac (SI) joint is a diarthrodial synovial joint. It is densely innervated by several levels of spinal nerves (L3-S1) and may produce lumbar disc-like symptoms when stimulated [14, 15].

ASIPP Systematic Review concludes that the evidence for intra-articular SI joint injections is limited for short (less than 6 weeks)- and long-term (6 weeks or longer) relief. The evidence for thermal and pulsed radiofrequency neurotomy in managing SI joint pain is limited.

Sympathetic Blocks

Stellate Ganglion Block

The stellate ganglion innervates the face, upper extremities, and heart. We block the stellate ganglion (see Fig. 9.2a, b) to treat sympathetically maintained pain (reflex sympathetic dystrophy or complex regional pain syndrome) of the upper extremity and face, frostbite, prolonged QT interval, hyperhidrosis, acute herpetic neuralgia, and angina. A stellate ganglion block involves injecting 10 cc of local anesthetic over the Chassaignac's tubercle on C-6 transverse process. This is usually done with the aid of fluoroscopic guidance in order to optimize outcomes. If patients experience significant pain relief following an injection (with no blockade of the motor and sensory fibers), we can determine that the pain is sympathetically maintained. In these cases, repeated blocks are frequently indicated to reduce pain.

Celiac Plexus Block

The celiac plexus innervates the upper abdominal viscera; thus, celiac plexus blocks (CPBs) can relieve pain originating from viscera in this area. Patients with

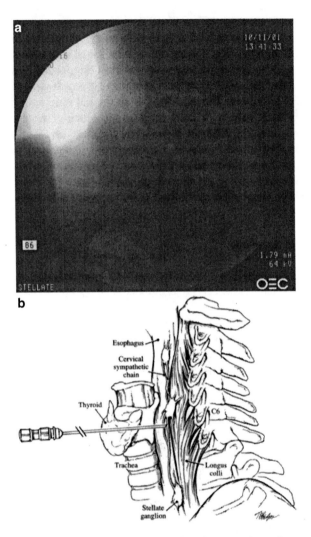

Fig. 9.2 Anteroposterior fluoroscopic view of needle placement for stellate ganglion block. Illustration of needle placement for stellate ganglion block

pain from upper abdominal malignancy, especially pancreatic cancer, as well as those with other forms of visceral disease, may benefit from a CPB [16] (see Fig. 9.3a, b). A successful CPB allows patients to reduce their consumption of analgesic drugs and, thus, reduce drug-related adverse effects. The diarrhea that is a common side effect of CPB usually resolves with conservative treatment. Many practitioners avoid CPB for nonmalignant pain because of the rare but catastrophic risk of causing a lumbar plexus injury and/or anterior spinal artery syndrome that can result in paraplegia.

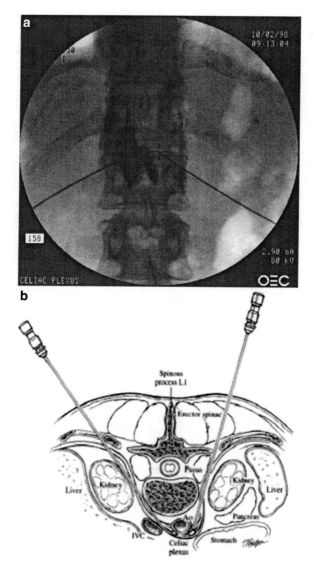

Fig. 9.3 Anteroposterior fluoroscopic view of needle placement for celiac plexus block. Illustration of needle placement for "classic" celiac plexus block

Lumbar Sympathetic Block

Lumbar sympathetic block (LSB) may be useful for treating sympathetically mediated pain of the lower extremities (see Fig. 9.4a, b). In patients with advanced peripheral vascular disease, for example, neurolytic or radiofrequency lesioning can lead to a 50% long-term improvement in blood flow, and relief of pain and ulceration. A phenol LSB can relieve pain and permit healing of gangrenous ulcers

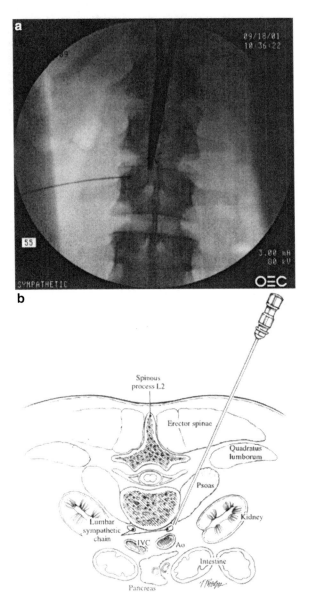

Fig. 9.4 Anteroposterior fluoroscopic view of needle placement for lumbar sympathetic block. Illustration of needle placement for lumbar sympathetic block

in diabetic patients, who experience pain upon resting, and in nondiabetic patients with digital gangrene or digital ulcers.

Superior Hypogastric Plexus Block

The superior hypogastric plexus innervates the pelvic area (Fig. 9.5a, b). Superior hypogastric plexus block (SHPB) can help patients who are suffering from pelvic

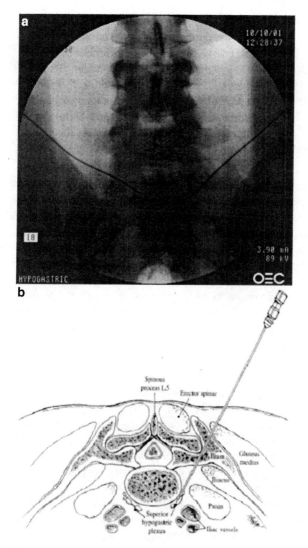

Fig. 9.5 Anteroposterior fluorosopic view of needle placement for superior hypogastric plexus block. Illustration of needle placement for superior hypogastric plexus block

pain arising from colon or cervical cancer [17]. If patients have extensive retro-peritoneal disease overlying the plexus, however, the neurolytic agent may be hindered from spreading appropriately to achieve the desired results [18]. Computed tomographic guidance and fluoroscopic guidance are useful techniques for administering SHPB to manage chronic pelvic pain in the presence of endometriosis. SHPB has also been used to treat severe chronic nonmalignant penile pain.

Ganglion Impar Block [19]

The ganglion impar is a solitary retroperitoneal structure located at the level of the sacrococcygeal junction that marks the termination of the paired paravertebral sympathetic chains. Blockade of the ganglion is used to manage intractable neo-plastic perineal pain of sympathetic origin [19].

Nerve Destruction

Neurodestruction has a prolonged effect and is generally reserved to treat cancer pain and certain spinal disorders. We use several techniques to destroy nerves.

Cryoablation can be accomplished by touching a nerve with a -60°C cryoprobe. This degenerates the nerve axons without damaging surrounding tissue. Nerves can also be destroyed by applying heat, phenol, or alcohol, or they can be cut with a surgical implement. With few exceptions, we destroy nerves only after we are satisfied that conservative therapies have failed to relieve pain.

Radiofrequency neuroablative procedures are generally performed on cervical, thoracic, and lumbar facet and sacroiliac joints and are among the most common tech-niques used in neuroablation. Some clinics use radiofrequency to treat chronic radicu-lar pain, complex regional pain syndrome, peripheral vascular disease, pancreatic disease, and trigeminal neuralgia. In 1996, for example, Lord et al. published the results of their double-blind, randomized, placebo-controlled trial of facet denervation for chronic cervicogenic pain [20]. They found marked reduction in pain in the group receiving denervation. Six of 12 patients in the control group (sham procedure) and 3 of 12 in the active-treatment group reported an immediate resumption of usual pain after the procedure or sham procedure. By 27 weeks, only one control patient versus seven active treatment patients were free of pain. Return to at least 50% of baseline pain occurred 263 days postprocedure in the active-treatment group and 8 days postprocedure in the control group, a statistically significant difference.

Chemical neurodestruction carries the risk of causing neuritis, which can be more painful than the original condition. The procedure is effective in 50–95% of patients. It can provide 3–6 months of significant pain relief. The complication rate associated with neurodestructive procedures is low in experienced hands.

Central Neurolysis

Intrathecal neurolysis is used to treat cancer pain limited to 2–3 dermatomes and to treat sacral pain. While this approach is much less common today, it can still be useful for patients with terminal diseases. A patient with pain on the left side due to cancer, for example, lies with the symptomatic side up for a hypobaric alcohol injection or with the symptomatic side down for a hyperbaric phenol injection.

Epidural scarring, fibrosis, and adhesions can be caused by postsurgical bleeding, leakage of nucleus pulposus contents into the epidural space, and repeated epidural or intrathecal procedures. The appearance of the scar tissue results from an inflammatory response and associated fibrocystic deposition. These adhesions can alter blood flow by disrupting epidural venous drainage and can increase swelling and nerve root edema – factors that can irritate nerve roots and cause pain.

A few techniques can be used to remove or reduce these adhesions. For example, the pathological segment of the epidural space can be accessed and a special epidural catheter passed into this space via an epidural needle. This polymer-coated, stainless steel catheter has a spiral tip. A commonly used catheter would include the Racz catheter. After insertion in the epidural space, the catheter is steered to the desired location. There are different ways to attain lysis at this point. Some practitioners believe that successful navigation of the catheter to the proper epidural location produces lysis of adhesions. It is also common to perform rapid injections of local anesthetics, with or without steroids, hyaluronidase, or plain saline into the epidural space to further lyse adhesions. The rapid injection of fluid itself may reduce scarring [21].

Intervention by entry into the epidural space, however, can lead to more scarring, and this possible outcome must be considered. Other risks include paralysis, bladder or bowel dysfunction, or unintentional subarachnoid or subdural injection of saline or local anesthetic.

Electrical Stimulation of the Spinal Cord and Peripheral Nerves

Centuries before we understood the nature of electricity, observant people discovered that electrical stimulation (caused by the proximity of electrical eels) relieved pain. When we learned to control electricity, healers replaced the eels with hand-cranked generators and continued to practice electrical therapy, without understanding how it relieved pain [22]. Eventually, in the mid-twentieth century, Melzack and Wall crafted a "gate-control theory of pain" that permitted the incorporation of electrical stimulation with modern medicine [23]. Now, despite our recognition of the shortcomings of this theory, we know that spinal cord stimulation (SCS) can effectively relieve pain [24], and multichannel, computerized systems with percutaneous electrodes allow us to stimulate the spinal cord, nerve roots, and peripheral nerves simultaneously (see Fig. 9.6a, b). In a review of experience with SCS during an 18-year period, North et al. found that at 7-year mean follow-up 52% of 171 patients with permanent implants reported at least 50% continued pain relief, with most also maintaining improvements in quality of life and reduced analgesic use [25]. The PROCESS trial demonstrated the efficacy of SCS in patients with failed back surgery syndrome (FBSS) as being superior to medication management alone [26]. North et al. compared reoperation with SCS to treat FBSS, using cross-ever as a primary outcome, and found that at 6-month follow-up, 67% of the 15 patients randomized for reoperation crossed over to SCS versus 17% of the 12 patients who received SCS at the outset [27].

In Europe, SCS is most often used to treat peripheral vascular disease in patients who can not undergo vascular reconstruction [28, 29]. In the USA, we use SCS

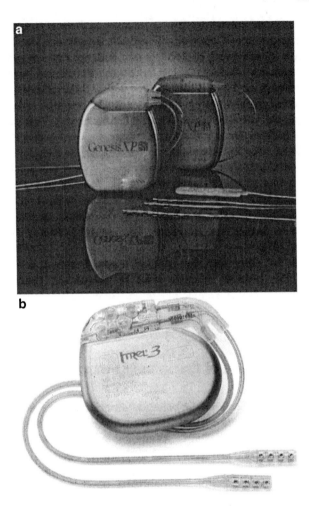

Fig. 9.6 Neuropulse generator and leads

most often to treat other conditions including radiculopathic pain arising from
FBSS [30].

Studies also validate the utility of SCS to treat complex regional pain syndrome
[31–33]. When Kemler et al. compared standard treatment for this syndrome with
SCS, they deemed SCS efficacious in 20 of the 24 SCS subjects and reported significant improvements in the SCS group compared with the 12 controls in the
standard treatment group [34].

In additional studies involving neuropathic pain, Harke et al. found that SCS
relieved pain in 23/28 patients with postherpetic neuralgia and 4/4 with acute herpes zoster [35], but Katayama et al. found that deep brain stimulation led to pain
control in six of ten patients (60%) with phantom limb pain; whereas, SCS was only
efficacious in 6 of 19 (34%) patients [36].

SCS is also an effective treatment for angina pectoris [37, 38], and the resulting paresthesia does not appear to interfere with signs of a myocardial infarction [39–41]. In a study of patients with angina treated by SCS for 6 weeks, the number of daily anginal episodes decreased from an average of 3.7–1.4, exercise duration increased, and mean ST-segment depression decreased, as did consumption of nitroglycerin [42]. Another study that employed Holter monitoring had similar results [43]. SCS, thus, can be considered a treatment for underlying heart disease.

Additional indications for SCS include pain associated with lumbar arachnoid fibrosis (arachnoiditis) [44] and spinal cord lesions with well-circumscribed segmental pain. Peripheral nerve stimulation is used to treat peripheral nerve injury [45], occipital neuralgia [46], incontinence [47], and pelvic and rectal pain [45].

Implantation of the SCS leads can result in dural puncture and/or infection (reported rates are 2–20%). If an infection involves deep tissue, the system must be temporarily removed. The mechanical system problems that can occur include electrode migration, connection leaks, or battery failure. Epidural hematoma or abscess, paralysis, and permanent nerve injury are among the rare serious complications of SCS.

SCS is an advanced pain therapy performed only when more conservative treatments fail [48]. With improvements in our techniques, equipment, and knowledge about which patients will benefit and how best to time the intervention to maximize success, we should be able to use SCS to treat pain arising from even more causes with even greater success [49]. To attain this goal, it is important to determine what causes the inconsistency of outcomes reported in the literature and to make the credentialing of implant physicians more rigorous.

ASIPP Systematic Review concludes that the evidence for SCS in FBSS and complex regional pain syndrome is strong for short-term relief and moderate for long-term relief.

Spinal Drug Delivery

During the past 15 years, the use of intraspinal drug delivery to treat chronic and cancer-related pain has increased. The use of implanted pumps for the long-term subarachnoid delivery of drugs is safe and efficacious. Selective spinal analgesia offers specific benefits, such as improved pain relief, improved lifestyle, and reduced side-effect profile, compared with an oral medical regime. Patients currently receiving oral medication who experience dose-limiting side effects and/or uncontrolled pain, for example, may be good candidates for intraspinal drug delivery. This could indicate acute injections of steroids or chronic infusions of analgesics via implanted pump.

Epidural Steroids

Mixter and Barr defined the herniated nucleus pulposus as a cause of pain radiating down the leg [50]. Lumbar epidurals for low back pain were introduced by Robecci and Capra in 1952 [51].

The epidural injection of corticosteroids has been used successfully to reduce nerve root irritation and inflammation. This injection can be performed in the neuraxis, where the injection bathes the spinal cord and neighboring nerve roots in the pathological area. Another approach is the transforaminal epidural injection (see Fig. 9.7). Here, the responsible nerve roots are identified and selectively targeted to receive epidural steroids. Patients with symptoms limited to specific nerve roots benefit from transforaminal epidural injections. One prospective, randomized study found a success rate of 84% after 1.4 years of treatment with transforaminal epidural steroid injections versus 48% after treatment with saline trigger point injections for lumbosacral radiculopathy arising from a herniated nucleus pulposus [52]. Similarly good results were reported for degenerative lumbar spinal stenosis, where 75% of 34 patients reported a 50% reduction in pain scores after an average of 1.9 injections [53].

Many studies have been performed to delineate the population that would be treated best with epidural steroid therapy. Abram and Hopwood, for example, have shown that the treatment of nonradicular pain that had persisted more than 24 months had a three-fold increase in failure of treatment. Factors that enhanced the possibility of a favorable outcome included pain of less than 6 months' duration, radiculopathy, and advanced patient education. Failure factors consisted of sleep disturbance, constant pain, and unemployment (secondary to the pain symptoms) [54, 55]. Sandrock and Warfield found that the positive outcome of epidural steroid injections is determined by successful diagnoses of nerve root inflammation, no history of surgery in the area, symptoms of short duration, younger patient age, and needle placement at the level of pathology [56]. There is obviously no consensus, but these results do indicate that outcome is related to nerve root irritation, recent onset of symptoms, and absence of psychological factors. Patients with herniated discs, spondylolisthesis, scoliosis, spinal stenosis (to a limited degree), and degenerative disc disease also seem to benefit.

ASIPP Systematic Review concludes that the evidence for caudal epidural steroid injections in managing chronic low back pain and radicular pain is strong for short-term relief and moderate for long-term relief. The evidence in postlumbar laminectomy syndrome and spinal stenosis is limited. Evidence indicates that interlaminar epidural steroid injections have strong short-term relief but limited long-term relief in the management of lumbar radiculopathy. There is strong evidence for short-term relief and limited for long-term relief with transforaminal epidural steroid injections in the management of lumbar radicular pain.

Intrathecal Therapy

Multiple spinal cord receptors and compounds play a role in the transmission of pain along various pathways to the brain. Pharmaceuticals can be administered to

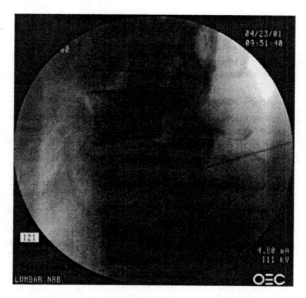

Fig. 9.7 Lateral fluoroscopic view of needle placement for transforaminal nerve root block

alter the behavior of some of these neurotransmitters, but we have not discovered the ideal agent or combination of agents to use in intrathecal pain therapy.

Preservative-free morphine and Ziconotide are the only analgesics approved for the intrathecal treatment of chronic pain by the US Food and Drug Administration (FDA).

In a series of 120 patients treated with intrathecal morphine for nonmalignant pain, Winkelmüller and Winkelmüller found that 92% of the patients were satisfied with the treatment, 81% reported improved quality of life, and 67% had pain reduction at 6-month follow-up [57]. In other large series, Paice et al. conducted a multicenter investigation involving 35 physicians and found that 95% of 429 patients (289 nonmalignant pain) had good to excellent results [58]. Smith and Staats performed a randomized controlled trial comparing intrathecal therapy to maximal medical therapy. They demonstrated that patients with cancer-related pain had a lower side-effect profile, lower pain scores and tended toward a longer life expectancy (Smith Staats et al.).

More recently, physicians have begun to use many other drugs intrathecally despite a lack of data on their neurotoxicity, their effect on pump stability, or their efficacy [59]. Numerous agents are widely used for cancer and non-cancer pain [60].

Multiple agents are considered safe and are used when morphine fails [61] (see Fig. 9.8). Some new agents such as Ziconotide, a synthetic neurotoxin based on the venom of a marine snail, may prove to be administrable only via the intrathecal route [62]. Prospective randomized controlled trials have demonstrated the effectiveness and safety of using Ziconotide to treat cancer pain and neuropathic pain [63].

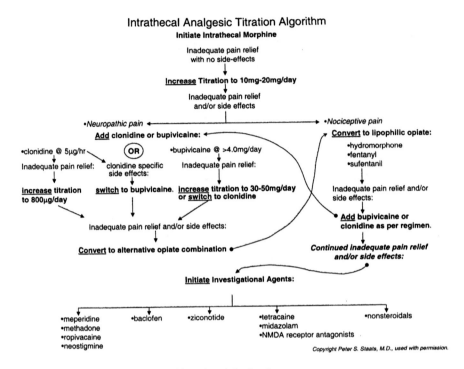

Fig. 9.8 Algorithm for Titration of Intrathecal Analgesics

Investigators are trying to determine to what degree pain treatment with intrathecal opioids enhances comprehensive medical management. In one randomized study, intrathecal therapy unexpectedly improved the survival of terminal cancer patients significantly, possibly by diminishing pain or by reducing the occurrence of drug toxicity [4]. Patients with cancer pain randomized to intrathecal therapy had a marked reduction in pain, toxicities, and, in fact, survival. Not only patients,but also family members (caregivers) reported improved quality of life.

Delivery Systems

Intrathecal drugs may be delivered, using a programmable pump or a constant rate spinal infusion pump, which is not programmable. The constant rate pump has only two basic variables: the size of the reservoir (which must be chosen before implantation) and the concentration of drug administered (which can be varied after implantation) (see Fig. 9.9a, b). The programmable pump, in contrast, allows clinicians to alter flow rate (see Fig. 9.9c). Unlike the programmable pump in which batteries must be replaced every 5–7 years, the constant rate spinal infusion pump does not require a battery. The larger reservoirs in constant rate pumps can lead to longer intervals between refills.

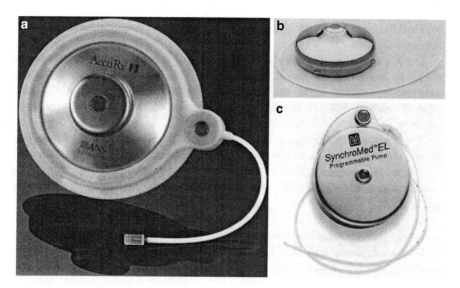

Fig. 9.9 Implantable pumps

ASIPP Systematic Review concludes that the evidence for implantable intrathecal infusion systems is strong for short-term improvement in pain of malignancy or neuropathic pain. The evidence is moderate for long-term management of chronic pain.

Vertebroplasty and Kyphoplasty

Vertebroplasty treats pain by treating the underlying condition of weak vertebrae. Thus, it involves injecting bond cement to create a permanent "cast" for vertebral structures damaged by osteoporotic compression fractures (its main use in the USA) [64], hemangiomas, or neoplasms (its main use in Europe) [65]. This procedure can lead to rapid pain relief.

Kyphoplasty expands vertebroplasty by first inflating a "balloon" in the vertebra to attempt to restore its height before injecting the cement [66, 67]. Some clinicians use kyphoplasty only to treat relatively fresh fractures – those that have had less than 2 weeks to heal [68].

Clinical experience indicates the promising nature of the expanded procedure. In 2001, [66] reported that preliminary results of a multicenter trial involving 376 procedures to treat 603 fractures in 340 patients showed a 90% improvement in symptoms and function [66]. That same year, Lieberman et al. published the results of 70 kyphoplasty procedures in 30 patients and noted that 47% of lost height was restored in 70% of the vertebral bodies treated. The investigators found that all outcome measures improved, and the only complications during the procedure were rib fractures in two patients and a pulmonary edema/myocardial infarction in another [67].

There is controversy about obtaining a venograph before vertebroplasty; some clinicians insist that this test improves safety [69], but others point out that the venography contrast agent can increase a patient's risk of a potentially fatal allergic reaction and can impede cement injection if the agent stagnates upon injection [70, 71].

The contraindications for vertebroplasty include a complete loss of vertebral height, the presence of osteoblastic metastasis, and acute fracture. The contraindications for kyphoplasty include bleeding disorders, fractured pedicles, the presence of solid tumors or osteomyelitis, and known allergy to the contrast agent used in the balloon.

In a controlled study of vertebroplasty without kyphoplasty, no advantage in pain relief was seen in comparison to controls [72]. Few controlled studies with or without kyphoplasty exist, yet it is agreed that vertebroplasty can cause serious neurologic complications. Thus, many clinicians recommend reserving these procedures for carefully selected subjects of clinical trials [73–75]. Initial follow-up studies, however, indicate that vertebroplasty may lead to long-term pain reduction and halt an otherwise likely progression to deformity. It is possible, on the other hand, that vertebroplasty may increase a patient's risk of another vertebral failure near the site of an original vertebroplasty repair [76].

The development and use of resorbable cements and kyphoplasty balloons will reduce the risk of these procedures and encourage their application in the USA to severe fractures [77, 78] and spinal malignancies [79].

ASIPP Systematic Review concludes that the level of evidence for success of vertebroplasty and kyphoplasty is moderate.

Intradiscal Electrothermal Annuloplasty and Nucleoplasty

The interior nucleus pulposus of a disc can bulge out of its tough outer annulus fibrosus, creating what is commonly known as a "herniation" and more properly called a "disc protrusion." When this protrusion compresses a nerve root, it can cause serious problems. Two new minimally invasive techniques, intradiscal electrothermal annuloplasty (IDET) and nucleoplasty were created to treat disc protrusions.

The theory behind IDET is that heat can modify the collagen and coagulate the pain nociceptors in the annulus of a disc. The exact mechanism of action of this procedure remains unknown, however. IDET is a 30-min outpatient procedure used to treat chronic, discogenic low back pain in patients who failed to respond to non-invasive treatment. In IDET, heat is delivered to the annulus via a specially designed electrode positioned in the outer circumference of a disc adjacent to the annulus fibrosus (see Fig. 9.10).

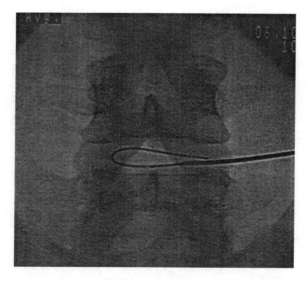

Fig. 9.10 Intradiscal Electrothermal Annuloplasty

Initial case reports in the literature indicate that the outcome of IDET is good for the first 6 months; the long-term effect remains unknown. In the first report of the clinical use of IDET, Saal and Saal found good results in 20 of 25 patients [80]. In a 12-month follow-up report on 36 IDET patients (with a convenience control sample of 17 patients whose insurers refused to cover IDET), Karasek and Bogduk noted that 32 IDET patients experienced "vigorous degrees of relief" at 3 months follow-up. Beyond this point, some deteriorated, while others continued to improve [81].

The contraindications of IDET have not yet been firmly established, but the criteria used to exclude subjects from trials include herniations larger than 4 mm, sequestered disc herniations (when pulposus material separates from the disc nucleus and floats in the spinal column), previous lower back surgery, vertebral canal stenosis, spondylolisthesis at the site, scoliosis, compression radiculopathy, pregnancy, and certain allergies. Complication rates have been low, but at least one report details the major complication of cauda equine syndrome [81].

Investigators developed the new technique of "radiofrequency discal nucleo-plasty" or "coblation nucleoplasty" after considering their experience with cobla-tion technology in other parts of the body in light of the well-established theory that the spine operates like a hydraulic system.

Using a straightforward technique and a standard radiofrequency generator, nucleoplasty is performed on an outpatient basis, with local anesthesia and fluoroscopic imaging [82]. The procedure involves inserting a "Spine Wand" into the disc (see Fig. 9.11) to apply radiofrequency to vaporize disc tissue, creating a channel (see Fig. 9.12), alternatively with thermal energy to coagulate the tissue and widen the channel. This process is repeated several times to create a cone-shaped hole in the herniated disc. The low temperatures (50–70°C) involved minimize

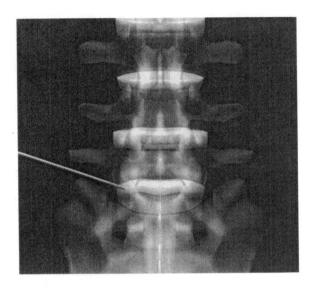

Fig. 9.11 Percutaneous Intradiscal Nucleoplasty

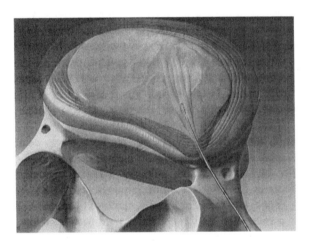

Fig. 9.12 Co-ablation channel made at 4:00 position

damage to surrounding tissue. Nucleoplasty may also eventually be used to treat disc extrusion (when pulposus tissue breaks through the annulus but remains attached to the nucleus) and, thus, may help more patients avoid surgery.

The exclusion criteria for nucleoplasty studies include sequestered herniation, contained herniation larger than one third the sagittal diameter of the spinal cord, stenosis, progressive neurological deficits, tumor, infection, and spinal fracture [83]. In the first report of clinical experience with nucleoplasty in 49 patients, the success rate was approximately 80% in the 40 with no previous spine surgery and less than 70% in the nine with previous spine surgery [84].

ASIPP Systematic Review concludes that the evidence for IDET in managing chronic discogenic low back pain is moderate. Nucleoplasty has been shown to provide limited short- and long-term relief.

Another thermal technique called Biaculoplasty is too new and has very few studies to be included in the review.

Percutaneous disc decompression can be considered with normal disc height and alignment. Advantages of this technique include less pain; less time missed from work and decreased scar tissue around the nerve roots when compared with open lumbar spine surgery.

MILD (minimally invasive lumbar decompression) is the first minimally invasive surgical treatment for lumbar spinal stenosis. The procedure involves the removal of bone or tissue causing pressure on the nerves through a minimally invasive approach, or a small puncture of the skin, about the diameter of a pencil. The minimally invasive nature of the procedure enables shorter inpatient stay and recovery compared to other open surgical treatment options such as laminotomy, laminectomy, and spinal fusion for lumbar spinal stenosis.

Botulinum Toxins

Botulinum toxins block or reduce muscle contractions and spasms by interfering with the release of acetylcholine, which transmits the contraction signal from the brain to muscle. Botulinum toxins may also block parasympathetic nervous system action.

Intramuscular injections of botulinum toxin performed on an outpatient basis three or four times per year are used to treat many conditions that involve abnormal muscle contraction. Hsiung et al. report that, during a 10-year period, they found substantial benefit in 63% of patients treated for cervical dystonia and 56% of those treated for writer's cramp [85]. When used for the treatment of whiplash, Botulinum toxin relieved pain significantly compared with a placebo treatment but showed a nonsignificant trend in improving subjective functioning [82]. In another study, 46 patients with coexisting chronic tension headaches and temporomandibular disorders reported a 50% or greater improvement in headache pain. A randomized, double-blind study found that 11/15 subjects who received Botulinum toxin A injections for low back pain had more than 50% pain relief versus 4/16 who received saline injections [84]. By 8 weeks, these figures were 9/15 and 2/16, and function had improved in the treatment group.

Contraindications to treatment with botulinum toxin include specific allergies, preexisting neuromuscular disease, consumption of blood thinners (including aspirin) and amino glycoside antibiotics, or other pharmaceuticals that interfere with neuromuscular transmission, dry eyes, everted lids (ectropion), pregnancy, lactation, and a history of reaction to the toxin. Botulinum toxins are not used in children under 12 years old.

The rare reports of death or significant debility or adverse cardiovascular events after botulinum toxin administration have not been definitively linked to the agent. If adverse effects, such as localized pain, tenderness, and/or bruising, occur, they are generally seen within a week of injection. These effects may be transient or may continue for several months. The expected action of the toxin is to induce weakness in the injected muscle(s); this weakness, however, may spread to adjacent muscles.

The therapeutic effect of a botulinum toxin injection lasts approximately 3 months and then diminishes gradually. Although botulinum toxins have been used for more than 10 years, we do not know the risks and benefits of long-term treatment.

Conclusion

Chronic pain may be difficult to diagnose, yet in order to develop the most appropriate therapeutic plan, one must make an accurate diagnosis. For example, all back pain is not the same. Some patients will respond to facet blocks, while others will respond to epidural steroids or require surgery. In still other patients, medical management will be most appropriate. When one understands the pathophysiology of a patient's pain, interventional therapies can be incorporated into the most appropriate therapeutic regimen.

References

1. Staats PS. The pain mortality link: unraveling the mysteries. In: Payne R, Patt R, Hill S, editors. Assessment and treatment of cancer pain. Seattle, WA: IASP Press; 1998. p. 145–56.
2. Staats PS, Sharma MC, Luthardt FW. Interventional strategies for pain management. In: Gloth M, editor. Handbook of pain relief in older adults: an evidence-based approach. Totowa, NJ: The Humana Press (in press).
3. Staats PS, Hekmat H, Sauter P, Lillemoe K. The effects of alcohol celiac plexus block, pain, and mood on longevity in patients with unresectable pancreatic cancer: a double-blind, randomized placebo-controlled study. Pain Med. 2001;2:28–34.
4. Smith TJ, Staats PS, Pool G, Deer T, Stearns L, Rauck R, et al. Randomized clinical trial of an implantable drug delivery system compared to comprehensive medical management for refractory cancer pain: impact on pain, drug-related toxicity, and survival. J Clin Oncol. 2002;20(19):4040–9.
5. WHO ladder
6. Cancer pain management: beyond the ladder. Grand Rounds, Cleveland Clinic Foundation, Cleveland, OH, April 1995.
7. Ashburn MA, Staats PS. The management of chronic pain. Lancet. 1999;353:1865–9.
8. Staats PS. Beyond the ladder. Journal of Back and Musculoskeletal Rehabilitation. 1998; 10(12):69–80.
9. Koes BW, Scholten RJ, Mens JM, Bouter LM. Efficacy of epidural steroid injections for low-back pain and sciatica: a systematic review of randomized clinical trials. Pain. 1995;63(3):279–88.
10. Loy TT. Epidural steroid injection for sciatica: an analysis of 526 consecutive cases with measurements and the whistle test. J Orthop Surg (Hong Kong). 2002;8(1):39–44.
11. Hopayian K, Mugford M. Conflicting conclusions from two systematic reviews of epidural steroid injections for sciatica: which evidence should general practitioners heed? Br J Gen Pract. 1999;49(438):57–61.

12. Carette S, Marcoux S, Truchon R, Grondin C, Gagnon J, Allard Y, et al. A controlled trial of corticosteroid injections into facet joints for chronic low back pain. N Engl J Med. 1991;1325(14):1002–7.

13. Boswell MV, Trescot AM, Datta S, Schultz DM, Hansen HC, Abdi S, et al. Interventional techniques: evidence based practice guidelines in the management of chronic spinal pain. Pain Physician. 2007;10(1):7–111.

14. Solonen KA. The sacroiliac joint in the light of anatomical, roentgenological and clinical studies. Acta Orthop Scand. 1957;27(Suppl):27.

15. Maigne JY, Aiviliklis A, Pfefer F. Results of sacroiliac joint double block and value of sacro-iliac pain provocation test in 4 patients with low back pain. Spine. 1996;2(16):1889–92.

16. . Staats PS [From my CV book chapter I wrote in on Pain Mortality link]

17. Plancarte R, Amescua C, Patt RB, Aldrete JA. Superior hypogastric plexus block for pelvic cancer pain. Anesthesiology. 1990;73(2):236–9.

18. Plancarte R, de Leon-Casasola OA, El-Helaly M, Allende S, Lema MJ. Neurolytic superior hypogastric plexus block for chronic pelvic pain associated with cancer. Reg Anesth. 1997;22(6):562–8.

19. Plancarte R, Amescua C, Patt RB, et al. Pre-sacral blockade of the ganglion of Walther (ganglion impar). Anesthesiology. 1990;73:A751.

20. Lord SM, Barnsley L, Wallis BJ, McDonald GJ, Bogduk N. Percutaneous radiofrequency neurotomy for chronic cervical zygapophyseal-joint pain. N Engl J Med. 1995;335(23):1721–6.

21. Manchikanti L, Staats PS, Singh V, Schultz DM, Vilims BD, Jasper JF, et al. Evidence-based practice guidelines for interventional techniques in the management of chronic spinal pain. Pain Physician. 2003;6:3–80.

22. Erb WT. Handbook of electro-therapeutics. Translated by L. Putzel. New York: W. Wood; 1883.

23. Melzack R, Wall PD. Pain mechanisms: a new theory. Science. 1965;150:971–8.

24. Krames E. Spinal cord stimulation: Indications, mechanism of action, and efficacy. Curr Rev Pain. 1999;3:419–26.

25. North RB, Kidd DH, Zahurak M, James CS, Long DM. Spinal cord stimulation for chronic, intractable pain: experience over two decades. Neurosurgery. 1993;32(3):384–94.

26. Kumar K, Talor RS, Jacques L, Eldabe S, Meglio M, Molet J, et al. Spinal cord stimulation versus conventional medical management for neuropathic pain: a multicenter randomized controlled trial in patients with failed back surgery syndrome pain. Pain. 2007;132(1–2):179–88.

27. North RB, Kidd DH, Lee MS, Piantodosi S. A prospective, randomized study of spinal cord stimulation versus reoperation for failed back surgery syndrome: initial results. Stereotact Funct Neurosurg. 1994;62:267–72.

28. Jivegard LE, Augustinsson LE, Holm J, Risberg B, Ortenwall P. Effects of spinal cord stimulation (SCS) in patients with inoperable severe lower limb ischaemia: a prospective randomized controlled study. Eur J Vasc Endovasc Surg. 1995;9:421–5.

29. Klomp HM, Spincemaille GHJJ, Steyerberg EW, et al. Spinal-cord stimulation in critical limb ischaemia: a randomized trial. Lancet. 1999;353:1040–4.

30. Bell GK, Kidd D, North RB. Cost-effectiveness analysis of spinal cord stimulation in treatment of failed back surgery syndrome. J Pain Symptom Manage. 1997;13:286–95.

31. Barolat G, Schwartzman R, Woo R. Epidural spinal cord stimulation in the management of reflex sympathetic dystrophy. Stereotact Funct Neurosurg. 1989;53:29–39.

32. Robaina FJ, Rodriguez JL, de Vera JA, Martin MA. Transcutaneous electric nerve stimulation and spinal cord stimulation for pain relief in reflex sympathetic dystrophy. Stereotact Funct Neurosurg. 1989;52:53–62.

33. Kemler MA, Reulen JPH, Barendse GAM, et al. Impact of spinal cord stimulation on sensory characteristics in complex regional pain syndrome type I. Anesthesiology. 2001;95:72–80.

34. Kemler MA, Barendse GAM, van Kleef M, de Vet HC, Rijks CP, Furnée CA, et al. Spinal cord stimulation in patients with chronic reflex sympathetic dystrophy. N Engl J Med. 2000;343:618–24.

35. Harke H, Gretenkort P, Ladleif HU, Koester P, Rahman S. Spinal cord stimulation in postherpetic neuralgia and in acute herpes zoster pain. Anesth Analg. 2002;94(3):694–700.
36. Katayama Y, Yamamoto T, Kobayashi K, Kasai M, Oshima H, Fukaya C. Motor cortex stimulation for phantom limb pain: comprehensive therapy with spinal cord and thalamic stimulation. Stereotact Funct Neurosurg. 2001;77(1–4):159–62.
37. de Jongste MJ, Hautvast RW, Hillege HL, et al. Efficacy of spinal cord stimulation as adjuvant therapy for intractable angina pectoris: a prospective, randomized clinical study. J Am Coll Cardiol. 1994;23:1592–7.
38. Murray S, Carson KG, Ewings PD, Collins PD, James MA. Spinal cord stimulation significantly decreases the need for acute hospital admission for chest pain in patients with refractory angina pectoris. Heart. 1999;82:89–92.
39. Andersen C, Hole P, Oxhoj J. Does pain relief with spinal cord stimulation for angina conceal myocardial infarction? Br Heart J. 1994;71(5):419–21.
40. Eliasson T, Jern S, Augustinsson LE, Mannheimer C. Safety aspects of spinal cord stimulation in severe angina pectoris. Coron Artery Dis. 1994;5(10):845–50.
41. Augustinsson LE, Eliasson T, Mannheimer C. Spinal cord stimulation in severe angina pectoris. Stereotactic Funct Neurosurg. 1995;65(1–4):136–41.
42. Hautvast RW, Blanksma PK, DeJongste MJ, et al. Effects of spinal cord stimulation on myocardial blood flow assessed by positron emission tomography in patients with refractory angina pectoris. Am J Cardiol. 1996;77(7):462–7.
43. De Jongste MJ, Haaksma J, Hautvast RW, Hillege HL, Meyler PW, Staal MJ, et al. Effects of spinal cord stimulation on myocardial ischemia during daily life in patients with severe coronary artery disease. A prospective ambulatory electrocardiographic study. Br Heart J. 1994;71(5):413–8.
44. Barolat G. Experience with 509 plate electrodes implanted epidurally from C1 to L1. Stereotact Funct Neurosurg. 1993;61(2):60–79.
45. Stojanovic MP. Stimulation methods for neuropathic pain control. Curr Pain Headache Rep. 2001;5(2):130–7.
46. Lou L. Uncommon areas of electrical stimulation for pain relief. Curr Rev Pain. 2000;4(5):407–12.
47. Jezernik S, Craggs M, Grill WM, Creasey G, Rijkhoff NJ. Electrical stimulation for the treatment of bladder dysfunction: current status and future possibilities. Neurol Res. 2002;24(5):413–30.
48. Deer TR. Current and future trends in spinal cord stimulation for chronic pain. Curr Pain Headache Rep. 2001;5:503–9.
49. Barolat G, Sharan AD. Future trends in spinal cord stimulation. Neurol Res. 2000;22:279–84.
50. Mixter WJ, Barr JS. Rupture of the intervertebral disc with involvement of the spinal canal. N Eng J Med. 1934;211:210–5.
51. Robecci A, Capra R. Hydrocortisone (compound F); first clinical experiments in the field of rheumatology. Minerva Med. 1952;43:1259–63.
52. Vad VB, Bhat AL, Lutz GE, Cammisa F. Transforaminal epidural steroid injections in lumbosacral radiculopathy: a prospective randomized study. Spine. 2002;27(1):11–6.
53. Botwin KP, Gruber RD, Bouchlas CG, Torres-Ramos FM, Sanelli JT, Freeman ED, et al. Fluoroscopically guided lumbar transforaminal epidural steroid injections in degenerative lumbar stenosis: an outcome study. Am J Phys Med Rehabil. 2002;81(12):898–905.
54. Hopwood MB, Abram SE. Factors associated with failure of lumbar epidural steroids. Reg Anesth. 1993;18:238.
55. Hopwood MB, Abram SE. What factors contribute to outcome with lumbar epidural steroids? In: Bond MR, Charlton JE, editors. Proceedings of the Sixth World Congress on Pain. Amsterdam: Elsevier Science Publishers; 1991.
56. Sandrock NJG, Warfield CA. Epidural steroids and facet injections. In: Principles and practice of pain management. New York: McGraw Hill; 1993.

57. Winkelmüller M, Winkelmüller W. Long-term effects of continuous intrathecal opioid treatment in chronic pain of nonmalignant origin. J Neurosurg. 1996;85:458–67.
58. Paice JA, Penn RD, Shott S. Intraspinal morphine for chronic pain: A retrospective, multicenter study. J Pain Symptom Manage. 1996;11:71–80.
59. Grabow TS, Derdzinski D, Staats PS. Spinal drug delivery. Curr Pain Headache Rep. 2001;5:510–5.
60. Deer T, et al. Clinical guidelines for intraspinal infusion: Report of an expert plan. Polyanalgesic Consensus Conference 2000. Bennett G et al. J Pain Symptom Manage 2000; 20(2):537–43.
61. Staats PS. Neuraxial infusion for pain control: when, why, and what to do after the implant. Oncology. 1999;13(5 Suppl 2):58–62.
62. Staats PS, Luthardt F, Shipley J, Jackson C, Fischer K. Long-term intrathecal ziconotide therapy: a case study and discussion. Neuromodulation. 2001;4:121–6.
63. Staats PS, Yearwood T, Charapata SG, Presley RW, Wallace MS, Byas-Smith M, et al. Intrathecal ziconotide in the treatment of refractory pain in patients with cancer or AIDS: a randomized controlled trial. JAMA. 2004;291(1):63–70.
64. Gangi A, Kastler BA, Dietemann JL. Percutaneous vertebroplasty guided by a combination of CT and fluoroscopy. Am J Neuroradiol. 1994;15:83–6.
65. Galibert P, Deramond H, Rosat P, Le Gars D. Preliminary note on the treatment of vertebral angioma by percutaneous acrylic vertebroplasty. Neurochirurgie. 1987;33:166–8.
66. Garfin SR, Yuan HA, Reiley MA. Kyphoplasty and vertebroplasty for the treatment of painful osteoporotic compression fractures. Spine. 2001;26:1511–5.
67. Lieberman IH, Dudeney S, Reinhardt M-K. Initial outcome and efficacy of "kyphoplasty" in the treatment of painful osteoporotic vertebral compression fractures. Spine. 2001;26(14):1631–8.
68. Mathis JM. Personal communication.
69. Hardouin P, Grados F, Cotton A, Cortet B. Should percutaneous vertebroplasty be used to treat osteoporotic fractures? An update. Joint Bone Spine. 2001;68(3):216–22.
70. Birkmeyer N. Point of view. Spine. 2001;26(14):1637–8.
71. Watts NB, Harris SDT, Genant HK. Treatment of painful osteoporotic vertebral fractures with percutaneous vertebroplasty or kyphoplasty. Osteoporosis Int. 2001;12(6):429–37.
72. Kallmes DF, Comstock BA, Heagerty PJ, Turner JA, Wilson DJ, Diamond TH, et al. A randomized trial of vertebroplasty for osteoporotic spinal fractures. N Engl J Med. 2009;361:569–79.
73. Grados F, Depriester C, Cayrolle G, Hardy N, Deramond H, Fardellone P. Long-term observations of vertebral osteoporotic fractures treated by percutaneous vertebroplasty. Rheumatology (Oxford) 2000;39(12):1410–4.
74. O'Brien JP, Sims JT, Evans AJ. Vertebroplasty in patients with severe vertebral compression fractures: a technical report. Am J Neuroradiol. 2000;21(8):1555–8.
75. Peh WC, Gilula LA, Peck DD. Percutaneous vertebroplasty for severe osteoporotic vertebral body compression fractures. Radiology. 2002;223(1):121–6.
76. Jensen ME, Kallmes DE. Percutaneous vertebroplasty in the treatment of malignant spine disease. Cancer J. 2002;8(2):194–206.
77. Saal JS, Saal JA. Management of chronic discogenic low back pain with a thermal intradiscal catheter. Spine. 2000;25:382–8.
78. Karasek M, Bogduk N. Twelve-month follow-up of a controlled trial of intradiscal thermal annuloplasty for back pain due to internal disc disruption. Spine. 2000; 25:2601–7.
79. Hsia AW, Isaac K, Katz JS. Cauda equina syndrome from intradiscal electrothermal therapy. Neurology. 2000;55:320.
80. Dworkin GE. Advanced concepts in interventional spine care. J Am Osteopath Assoc. 2002;102(9 Suppl 3):S8–11.
81. Sharps LS, Isaac Z. Percutaneous disc decompression using nucleoplasty. Pain Physician. 2002;5:121–6.

82. Freund BJ, Schwartz M. Treatment of whiplash associated neck pain [corrected] with botulinum toxin-A: a pilot study. J Rheumatol. 2000;27(2):481–4.
83. Sharps IZ. Percutaneous disc decompression using nucleoplasty. Pain Physician. 2002;5:121–6.
84. Foster L, Clapp L, Erickson M, Jabbari B. Botulinum toxin A and chronic low back pain: a randomized, double-blind study. Neurology. 2001;56(10):1290–3.
85. Hsiung GY, Das SK, Ranawaya R, Lafontaine AL, Suchowersky O. Long-term efficacy of Botulinum toxin A in the treatment of various movement disorders over a 10-year period. Mov Disord. 2002;17(6);1288–93.

Chapter 10
Pain Management in Long-Term Care

Susan L. Charette and Bruce A. Ferrell

The importance of pain control in the geriatric patient population is now well recognized and has received increasing attention over the past 20 years. Growing interest and commitment by the medical community has lead to an advancing body of research and literature in this area. Nursing home patients represent a large and distinctive subset of the geriatric population whose pain issues have been previously overlooked. With the aging of the population, more elderly patients will reside in nursing homes in the future and estimates project that the number of nursing home residents will likely rise to greater than 5 million by the year 2040 [1]. In addition, it has been reported that 43% of adults 65 years and older will enter a nursing home some time before they die [2]. Some patients will stay only short term, while others will remain for years. Along with the expected increase in the nursing home population, the demographics are expected to change and include older and more disabled patients in the future [3].

In the long-term care setting, pain is underdiagnosed, underreported, and undertreated by physicians and nursing staff. Patient care typically focuses on the management of underlying medical problems, and pain is usually not viewed as a primary endpoint [4]. However, the presence of pain is a negative influence that can affect patients at multiple levels. Impaired mobility, decreased socialization, depression, sleep disturbances, and increased health utilization and costs have been associated with pain [5–7]. In addition, a number of geriatric conditions may be exacerbated by pain including deconditioning, gait impairment, falls, slow rehabilitation, polypharmacy, cognitive dysfunction, and malnutrition [8]. Thus, quality of life and functional status may be adversely affected without the adequate assessment and management of pain.

Pain assessment and management in nursing home patients present a unique set of challenges. The nursing home environment is variable and settings range from

S.L. Charette (✉)
UCLA Division of Geriatrics, 200 UCLA Medical Plaza, Suite 420,
Los Angeles, CA 90095, USA
e-mail: scharette@mednet.ucla.edu

F.M. Gloth, III (ed.), *Handbook of Pain Relief in Older Adults: An Evidence-Based Approach*, Aging Medicine, DOI 10.1007/978-1-60761-618-4_10,
© Springer Science+Business Media, LLC 2011

subacute, skilled nursing units to long-term, custodial facilities. Nursing home patients are a heterogeneous group and their goals of care vary. Some may undergo rehabilitation with the goal of going home, while others may receive end-of-life care for a terminal condition, and many will be admitted for long-term, custodial but not necessarily terminal care. The number of beds, staffing ratios, and supportive services differ widely between nursing homes. The nursing home is a "low tech" environment with limited resources. Most lack the ancillary services that are offered in the acute setting such as in-house pharmacies and radiology services. One-on-one care is provided for the most part by nursing assistants under the supervision of a charge nurse, and staff-to-patient ratios may vary from as high as 1:6 to lower than 1:20. In addition, registered nurses may not be scheduled for every shift, and intravenous medications and other treatments are often not available around-the-clock. Unlike in the acute setting, physician visits are typically monthly or occasionally when an acute event occurs. Thus, physicians may not be aware of changes in a patient's condition, symptoms, or pain occurrences. Consultants such as neurologists, anesthesiologists, and pain specialists do not routinely visit nursing homes and may be reluctant to provide consultation services in this setting.

This chapter will provide a brief overview of pain in long-term care. The first section will focus on the epidemiology of pain in the nursing home followed by a discussion of the barriers to assessment and management of pain in this population. Guidelines for the assessment and management of pain will be outlined. The chapter will conclude with recommendations for quality improvement in the nursing home.

Epidemiology of Pain in the Nursing Home

Pain is a frequent complaint of older patients and a common problem in the nursing home. Most cross-sectional studies have demonstrated that the overall prevalence of pain rises with advancing age, although this increase does not appear to continue beyond the seventh decade [9]. Why is there a greater prevalence of pain in older patients? Researchers have investigated whether there may be changes in pain perception and altered pain reporting in older patients, and the data are inconclusive [10]. "Pathological load" – an increase in medical conditions causing pain – is probably the primary factor behind the increase in pain complaints with advancing age [9]. Nursing home patients tend to have more medical problems and medications than their community-dwelling counterparts. A study of 217 subjects from ten nursing facilities found an average of eight active medical problems and nine medications per patient [7].

While the prevalence of pain in community-dwelling older patients is about 25–50%, the prevalence of pain in the nursing homes has been documented to be as high as 45–80% [4, 5, 9, 11–18]. The prevalence variability across studies is multifactorial and cannot be entirely explained by review of the data. Potential reasons for this variability include number of subjects in each group, assessment tools used, questions asked, and patients' cognitive status [9].

Knowledge of the type and source of pain is necessary for effective pain assessment and management. In a study of 97 subjects from a large long-term care facility, 71% of the patients had at least one pain complaint – 34% of whom had continuous pain and 66% had intermittent pain [5]. Of those with intermittent pain, 51% reported daily symptoms. Table 10.1 lists most common sources of pain which are musculoskeletal including lower back pain, arthritis, and previous fracture sites followed by neuropathic pain syndromes and malignancies [5, 7]. Other less common but significant causes of persistent pain are claudication, headache, and leg cramps [4].

Pain affects quality of life. Pain in nursing home residents may be associated with impaired mobility, sleep disturbance, and a reduced ability to enjoy recreational activities [5, 17]. Loss of function increases with the severity of the underlying pain [17]. Other research has shown a strong correlation between pain and depression in nursing home residents even after controlling for functional status and physical health [6]. The impact of pain on physical and psychological functioning may influence the disposition and long-term outcomes for nursing home residents.

Table 10.1 Sources of pain

Source	Frequency
Low-back pain	26 (40%)
Previous fractures	9 (14%)
Neuropathies	7 (11%)
Leg cramps	6 (9%)
Knee, arthritic	6 (9%)
Claudication	5 (8%)
Shoulder, arthritic	5 (8%)
Foot	5 (8%)
Hip, arthritic	4 (6%)
Neck	4 (6%)
Headache	4 (6%)
Generalized pain	3 (5%)
Neoplasm	2 (3%)
Angina	2 (3%)
Eye	1 (1%)
$N = 65$	

(Numbers total more than 100% because some
   subjects had more than one source of pain)

Source: Ferrell BA, Ferrell BR, Osterweil D. Pain in the nursing home. J Am Geriatr Soc.1990;38:412; with permission

The epidemiology of pain may be influenced by how pain has been measured. Typically, pain is either assessed by patient self-report or nursing assessment. Multiple studies have used the Minimum Data Set (MDS), which collects multiple data points including those on patients' pain as recorded by the nursing home staff. These studies have shown a lower prevalence of pain among nursing home patients in the range of 20–41% [14, 19–21]. It has been generally felt and recently documented that MDS documentation underestimates the frequency and intensity of pain when compared with patients' reports [14, 22]. Nursing aides, who typically work closely with a group of patients, appear to be more accurate at assessing pain intensity than licensed practical nurses [22].

The prevalence of pain is even lower in nursing home patients with cognitive impairment. In a study of over 500 nursing home patients, chart abstraction demonstrated that reports of pain decreased as cognitive abilities declined [21]. Nurses completing the MDS reported pain prevalence of 34, 31, 24, and 10%, respectively, for nursing home residents with no, mild, moderate, and severe cognitive impairment ($P < 0.001$) [21]. Another study compared a pain questionnaire completed by certified nursing assistants with documentation in the MDS for cognitively impaired patients [20]. The questionnaires reported a greater prevalence of pain than the MDS (40 vs. 20%) [20]. Cognitively impaired patients are difficult to assess and often suffer from medical conditions that cause pain. Current reporting underestimates the presence of pain in this subset of the nursing home population.

Physicians have also been shown to underestimate nursing home resident pain [12, 16]. In a study by Sengstaken and King, 66% of communicative patients were described as having chronic pain and treating physicians did not detect this problem in a third of these residents [12]. A large study including over 30 nursing homes found that almost 50% of cognitively intact patients reported chronic pain; however, nearly half of these patients had no physician assessment of pain in the past year [16].

Pain management strategies in the nursing home are often limited in scope and only partially successful in controlling pain [7]. In a large, cross-sectional study of nursing home patients with cancer, more than a quarter of patients in daily pain did not receive any analgesia [19]. This same study found that age over 85, minority race, cognitive impairment, and number of other medications received were independent predictors of failure to receive analgesia [19]. Other research has shown that many patients receiving pain medication still complain of pain and suggests that the effectiveness of pain management must frequently be assessed [12].

There is a wide range of pharmacologic treatment options available for the management of pain. In a study of more than 20,000 nursing home patients, the most common analgesics were acetaminophen (37.2%), propoxyphene (18.2%), hydrocodone (6.8%), and tramadol (5.4%) [23]. Less than half of all analgesics were given as standing doses, and acetaminophen was usually prescribed as needed (65.6%), at doses less than 1,300 mg per day [23]. Nonsteroidal anti-inflammatory drugs (NSAIDs) were prescribed as a standing dose more than 70% of the time, and one-third of NSAIDs were prescribed at high dose [23]. This large study shows that the type, dose, and frequency of pain medications ordered in the nursing home are often inadequate and inappropriate.

Barriers to Successful Pain Assessment and Management in the Nursing Home Patient

Effective pain assessment and management in nursing home patients is challenging. This special setting and patient population present a number of unique obstacles and problems that must be addressed. These barriers exist at several levels and include patient, facility, nursing, and physician factors.

There are multiple patient-based issues that make pain assessment and management difficult to carry out in the long-term care setting. Most nursing home patients have multiple medical problems. Pain may be overshadowed by these other issues and given a lower priority when it is identified. Visual, hearing, and motor impairments are common and can make assessment more difficult [4]. Patients may not report their symptoms for a variety of reasons. Some may feel that those around them are worse off than themselves, while others may expect pain to be a natural part of aging and not worth reporting [5]. Some patients cite stoicism as a reason for not seeking pain medication when in pain [24]. Nursing home residents often try to avoid being labeled a "complainer" because of the negative effects this might have on their overall care [5, 25]. Often they fear pain and what it represents – more tests, loss of autonomy, worsening disease, and possibly death [25]. They may also have concerns about medication side effects and the potential for addiction [24]. These resident preferences and beliefs may lead to declined pain interventions regardless of the staff's motivation to make the resident more comfortable [24].

Cognitive impairment presents a specific challenge that is commonplace in the nursing home. It is estimated that over 65% of nursing home residents have cognitive impairment or mental illness [7]. In a large study of ten community-based nursing homes, 21% of the patients were mute or unresponsive and unable to make their needs known [7]. Of the subjects who did complain of pain, 17% could not complete any of the quantitative assessment scales presented, although they were able to give some form of a qualitative description of pain. Impaired older people who retain communication skills are usually able to report experienced pain when asked, however, as cognitive impairment increases, reported problems with pain decrease [26]. A study of hospitalized hip fracture patients demonstrated that demented patients received one-third the amount of morphine sulfate as compared to the cognitively intact patients, even though their situations and potential for pain were similar [27].

Barriers to pain assessment and management may exist among nurses and other staff members who are at the frontline of patient care in the nursing home. Specific staff-related challenges may include staff's knowledge and ability to recognize and treat pain, communication between the nursing aides and the charge nurse, and level of familiarity with a resident's daily habits and behavior patterns [28]. Nurses may have fears about giving pain medication to elderly patients, misconceptions about addiction, and hesitancy to provide medication when it is appropriate [28]. In particular, they may be apprehensive about potential adverse effects of pain medication such as constipation, sedation, and falls [29]. When patients are thought to be using complaints of pain to get attention or felt to be too demanding, these perceptions may have a negative effect on the nurse–patient relationship and ultimately the diagnosis and treatment of pain [28]. On the other hand, many nurses become very close to their patients in this setting and advocate for good pain management.

Physicians also face a number of challenges when it comes to assessing and managing pain in the nursing home. For starters, many doctors leave training with only minimal exposure to patient care in the nursing home setting. In a recent study, more than 30% of senior internal medicine residents felt ill-equipped to care for nursing home patients [30]. Primary care physician training in pain assessment and management is often limited and over one-quarter of senior internal medicine residents felt inadequately prepared to manage pain [30]. Many geriatric medicine training programs also lack a focused curriculum in pain management, and geriatricians may complete their fellowship with little exposure to this area, even though it is an expected area of expertise [31]. Physicians underestimate pain in patients, whether they are cognitively intact or impaired, and elderly patients often receive inadequate analgesia [12, 27]. Specifically physicians do poorly when it comes to the assessment of pain, performing targeted history and physical examinations, documenting risk factors for the use of analgesics, and documenting response to treatment [16]. Physicians clearly have limitations in their ability to identify and treat pain, and these may relate to deficiencies in knowledge and experience as well as concerns regarding the management of opioid side effects, the possibility of addiction, and the risk of delirium [27].

In addition to the challenges presented by patients and the healthcare providers, there are specific nursing home barriers that complicate pain assessment and control in this setting. First, there are often logistical difficulties in carrying out diagnostic procedures at the facility – for example, radiology services are usually not available on site and must be provided through portable services. Such services are often delayed and inferior to the more sophisticated, fixed equipment. Transportation of nursing home residents off-site may create additional hardships and discomfort, thus making some diagnostic techniques less feasible. Second, advanced management techniques (e.g. epidural injections) are typically unavailable and consultants (e.g. anesthesiologists) do not routinely visit nursing homes. Finally, additional limitations may arise once pain management has been ordered due to restricted formularies by insurance companies, the need for special prescriptions for narcotic pain relievers, and constraints in pharmacy service availability.

Recognizing these challenges is an important part of managing pain in the nursing home. Patients should be asked routinely about pain and reassured that their concerns are important and valid. Their questions about the meaning of pain, necessary tests, and side effects of medications need to be answered. For those who are unable to communicate or have significant cognitive impairment, the patient's family or primary decision maker should be included in the assessment and plan. Education and training of nurses and physicians in the treatment of pain, particularly as it relates to older adults and the long-term care environment, are crucial. These issues have received increasing attention over the last few years and hopefully nursing homes will be better equipped to meet these challenges in the future. The next sections will describe effective pain assessment and management strategies for nursing home patients and offer practical methods for overcoming these barriers.

Assessment of Pain in the Nursing Home

The assessment of pain in the nursing home should begin with the initial intake on admission. The nursing staff typically performs a detailed evaluation on every patient who enters a nursing home. In addition, a complete history and physical examination by the patient's physician provides an opportunity to identify pertinent diagnoses and concerns, current and past treatments, and problems to be addressed. Subsequent assessments should be performed when there is a change in the level of care, after a pain intervention, and as part of the MDS [32]. The interdisciplinary team is an integral part of patient management in the nursing home and is composed of representatives from nursing, social services, rehabilitation therapy, and dietary services [32]. Other personnel, e.g., the activities coordinator, may also be included. The team generates problem-based care plans for each patient and these are revised every 30–90 days depending on the patient's level of care [32]. Starting with the day of admission, there are multiple opportunities for the on-going assessment of pain in the nursing home.

The goal of an assessment is to find out if a patient has pain, characterize it, determine its etiology, and determine the best mode of treatment. What is the best way to assess pain in the nursing home? Most elderly nursing home residents, including those with mild-to-moderate cognitive impairment, are able to report, if they have pain when asked [7, 13, 26]. Many patients with more advanced cognitive impairment are able to report on their pain if asked simple, concrete, yes or no questions. Patients' self report of pain may be more dependable than nurses' impressions. In a study of 45 pairs of nursing home patients and their regular nursing aides, each was asked to describe the prevalence, location and intensity of the patient's pain and only one third of the pairs were in agreement [33]. These results demonstrate that patient self-report is more reliable than observer assessment and reinforce the importance of talking with patients about their symptoms and taking their pain complaints seriously.

As part of the Omnibus Budget Reconciliation Act of 1987, the Resident Assessment Instrument (RAI) with its MDS was developed to improve patient care through systematic patient care planning. The MDS evaluates residents for a range of nursing home quality measures including pain and is performed on every resident at a facility that receives federal funding under Medicare or Medicaid. The data points are typically entered by a member of the nursing staff who uses a variety of sources of information – the resident, facility staff, the resident's physician, and the medical chart – to determine the most appropriate response for each item [34]. The results of the MDS are forwarded electronically to the state and to the Department of Health and Human Services. The MDS section on pain, shown in Table 10.2, records the "highest level of pain present in the last 7 days" in terms of the frequency with which the "resident complains or shows evidence of pain" (0 = no pain, 1 = less than daily, and 2 = daily) and the intensity of pain (1 = mild pain, 2 = moderate pain, and 3 = times when pain is horrible or excruciating). Direct

Table 10.2 Minimum Data Set 2.0 Pain Items

Pain symptoms (Code the *highest level of pain* present in the *last 7 days*)

1. *Frequency* with which resident complains or shows evidence of pain
   (a) No pain (*skip to J4*)
   (b) Pain less than daily
   (c) Pain daily
2. *Intensity* of pain
   (a) Mild pain
   (b) Moderate pain
   (c) Times when the pain is horrible or excruciating (To be determined by nursing staff based
       on patient report and nursing assessment)

Source: MDS Medicare PPS Assessment Form from the Center for Medicare and Medicaid
Services Website (http://cms.hhs.gov/medicaid/mds20/mpaf.pdf)

measures of pain frequency and intensity have been shown to be good predictors of
patients' own pain rating on the Visual Analogue Scale (VAS) [34]. The results of
the MDS may be a useful source of information on patient pain as this assessment
is performed on every new patient, when there is a change in condition, and quar-
terly. Unfortunately research has shown that the MDS underdocuments the prevalence of patient pain, particularly in patients with cognitive impairment [20, 21].
Nurses and other staff members completing the MDS may not be able to identify
signs of pain in those who are unable to report it [34]. The 3.0 version of the MDS
awaits real world evaluation to see whether modifications to the pain component
will prove more representative.

A variety of pain assessment tools are available and many can be easily implemented in the nursing home setting. At the simplest level, patients can be asked
if they have pain and then questioned further regarding its quality, intensity, and
location. Such questions can easily be posed with the passing of medications or
at the time of vital sign measurements. For purposes of recording the level of
pain, capable patients should be asked to rate their pain on a scale of zero to five
or zero to ten. Other potential tools include the pain thermometers, verbal
descriptor scales, numerical scales, the faces pain scales, and functional pain
scales. Further discussion of the merits of some of these scales occurs in Chap. 2.
These instruments are widely used and can be incorporated into pain assessment
protocols. Ultimately, pain assessment instruments must be practical, easy to
administer, and reliable.

The assessment of pain in patients with cognitive impairment is challenging. This
is especially true for patients with advanced dementia who are noncommunicative
and unable to report when they have pain. The lower prevalence of pain among cognitively impaired nursing home residents may be related to such difficulties with pain
assessment. A growing body of research has focused on the behaviors of patients with
moderate-to-advanced dementia as a means for pain evaluation and an increasing
number of assessment tools for the cognitively impaired have been developed and
studied over the past 5 years [29, 35]. A study of nurses' perceptions of pain in
patients with dementia found a core group of behaviors that might be indicators of

pain including specific physical repetitive movements, vocal repetitive behaviors, physical signs of pain, and changes in behavior from the norm [28]. Several assessment tools have been developed to assess for behaviors and patient features that might be associated with pain in patients with advanced dementia, including the Discomfort Scale and the Assessment of Discomfort in Dementia [36, 37]. The MDS has also been suggested as a useful instrument for the cognitively impaired because it does not rely on patient self-report [13]. However, a recent study demonstrated that a three-item pain questionnaire administered to certified nursing assistants was a more sensitive measure of pain and more strongly associated with analgesic use than the MDS [20]. Whether using a specially designed instrument or monitoring for specific behaviors, nursing aides, family members, and other caregivers are generally able to offer useful insight on pain in cognitively impaired patients.

For all nursing home patients, pain assessment should evaluate the impact of the pain on quality of life and function. Pain may cause significant functional limitations including mobility, sleep, appetite, and psychosocial function [38]. Knowledge of these functional deficits is helpful as this may be the underlying reason for a short stay or long-term admission, and pain may be a modifiable and secondary factor [38]. The pain experience can be influenced by a range of variables – medical, psychosocial, cognitive, neuropsychological, and behavioral – and patient evaluations should taken into account the impact of pain in these domains [38].

When physicians evaluate pain in the nursing home patients, conferring with staff members and a review of the chart are a good place to start. Talking with and observing the patient can be extremely informative. Often a little extra time is needed to get the details but is well worth it. Inherent to the assessment process, physicians need to take time to make the patient comfortable, adjust their glasses and hearing aids, reduce environmental distractions, and use repetition and validating questions to help establish the accuracy of response [39]. Physical examination should focus on the musculoskeletal and nervous system as problems in these systems are so common [4]. In particular, evaluation for trigger points, straight leg raise, joint range of motion, and autonomic, motor and sensory deficits should be considered [4]. When a new complaint of pain is reported, patients should undergo an assessment and the pain should not be attributed to a preexisting illness [4]. The patient's prior and current functional status should be determined, and his or her performance with physical therapy and occupational therapy should be reviewed. Functional status is an important outcome measure for pain management in order to ensure that mobility and independence are maximized [4]. In addition, depression is commonly associated with pain and should be addressed at the time of the assessment [6].

Pain Management in the Nursing Home

Little attention or research has focused on the management of geriatric pain, especially among nursing home patients [4]. A comprehensive, interdisciplinary approach to pain management – including medications as well as nonpharmaceutical modalities – is ideal. Analgesic medications are the most common strategy for pain management in the nursing home setting [5]. Those with the lowest side-effect profile should be selected initially, as these patients are at high risk for adverse reactions due to their various medical problems and need for multiple medications [4]. Polypharmacy is common and potential drug–drug interactions must be considered with the addition of each new medication.

Initiating pain management in the nursing home can be challenging. As mentioned previously, most long-term care facilities do not have a pharmacy on the premises and it may take hours to get medication orders filled by outside pharmacies. Nursing homes are potential sites of drug diversion and abuse, and most states do not allow them to keep a contingency supply of opioids [39]. State regulations may require special prescriptions by physicians for opioids, and pharmacies may not stock certain narcotics. These and other factors may make effective treatments difficult to obtain. When dosing opioids in this population, it is important to remember that older patients may be more sensitive to the analgesic properties of these medications. Smaller doses may be adequate and it is best to start low and increase slowly [15]. Potential side effects include drowsiness, delirium, and respiratory depression, especially in opioid-naïve patients. Tolerance does develop over time and patients experience decreased drowsiness and respiratory depression with prolonged use. While oral opioid formulations are typically adequate, some patients may require parenteral dosing, often by continuous infusion. Many nursing homes may not have staff who are familiar and skilled in the administration of parenteral opioids and related devices (e.g. CADD® pumps), and this may restrict or limit the usefulness of these modalities. Subcutaneous, sublingual, or transdermal dosing may provide effective alternatives, if intravenous therapy is not available and oral medications are not an option. Additionally, there are often agencies that can provide nursing consultants and services in many communities to assist with pain management including parenteral therapies.

A major limitation in the use of analgesia for pain management is the increased risk and incidence of side effects in older patients. NSAIDs are associated with gastrointestinal side effects including gastritis and GI upset. Many of these patients have multiple risk factors for GI bleeding including multiple organ insufficiency, need for concomitant anticoagulant therapy, and preexisting history of upper and lower GI bleeds [39]. Other NSAID-related side effects seen in elderly patients include renal impairment, hypertension, bleeding, headaches, confusion, edema, and constipation. A recent review suggests that traditional NSAIDs should probably not be used in this population, especially in high doses for long periods [15].

Adjuvant medications may be especially useful in certain conditions. Tricyclic antidepressants and anticonvulsants are primary treatment options for neuropathic pain from herpes zoster, diabetic neuropathy, and peripheral neuropathy. However, their side effect profile must be considered before dosing in this population. The tricyclic antidepressants can cause significant anticholinergic effects and gabapentin, the most commonly used anticonvulsant for neuropathic pain, is associated with somnolence and ataxia. Two newer agents, pregabalin, an anticonvulsant similar to gabapentin, and duloxetine, a selective serotonin and norepinephrine reuptake inhibitor, have been FDA-approved for the treatment of neuropathic pain as well as fibromyalgia. The 5% lidocaine patch is an alternative for the management of pain from postherpetic neuralgia. Several studies have suggested the potential usefulness of miacalcin on reducing bone pain due to osteoporotic fractures [40]. Local application of capsaicin cream may provide some relief for patients with arthritis and neuropathies.

It is worth mentioning that vitamin D deficiency, a prevalent problem in the nursing home population, has been associated with pain related to increased rates of fracture, osteomalacia, and vitamin D deficiency pain syndrome [41–43]. Because of the ease of treatment with Vitamin D_3 megadosing (50,000–100,000 IU by mouth) every month, it is a potential cause of pain that should not be overlooked.

When prescribing pain medications in the nursing home, it is necessary to pay close attention to dosing orders. As discussed previously, patients may not ask for pain medications for a variety of reasons, and those with cognitive impairment may not be able to [16, 21]. Standing orders should be used for patients who have constant or chronic pain, or symptoms occurring at certain times of the day, such as before physical therapy. In addition, the patient and staff should be queried routinely about the adequacy of the medication regimen, the need frequency for PRN doses, and presence of side effects. The medication administration record (MAR) should be reviewed at the time of patient visits. The MAR documents current patient medications, missed doses, and PRN doses given, and may also list experienced side effects and vital sign measurements. This information along with input from the patient and staff will allow for optimal pain management.

Nonpharmacologic approaches, used alone or in combination with appropriate analgesic medications, are an integral part of pain management in the nursing home. In-house physical therapy offers patient-specific programs emphasizing flexibility, strengthening, and conditioning as well as other treatments such as local massage, stretching, ice and heat treatments, and ultrasound [44]. Transcutaneous electrical nerve stimulation (TENS) can be a useful adjunct in the management of pain, especially for patients with chronic neuropathy and postfracture recovery [45]. While nondrug approaches are appealing, there are limitations to their effective implementation. Many nursing homes hire out physical therapists, and patients may not have their own, regular therapist who is in charge and familiar with the goals and plan of treatment. Heating pads are often not hot enough due to justified concerns over risk of thermal injury, ultrasound may not be available, and the time allocated may be insufficient for the therapist to use multiple modalities. Finally, other interventions such as relaxation, behavioral therapy, and acupuncture are usually unavailable in the nursing home setting

Hospice should be considered in appropriate patients. Patients receiving hospice care have been shown to have better analgesic management of daily pain and are more likely to receive pain medications consistent with the current guidelines [46]. While hospice offers the nursing home patient additional support services and pain management expertise, it removes a degree of responsibility from the nursing home staff. Clinicians should be aware that potential conflicts can occur when lines of authority and responsibility for patient care are fragmented [39].

There are some patients that may require treatment beyond the scope of the nursing home physician and staff. Patients with problems with long-standing pain or substance abuse may benefit from a specialist with appropriate expertise [15]. Other patients may need interventions not available at the nursing home, such as an epidural by an anesthesiologist, and require evaluation and treatment at an outside office or facility. While these special circumstances exist, there are multiple treatment options available in the nursing home, and, with their addition to patient care, effective pain management is possible.

Quality Improvement in the Nursing Home

Pain assessment and management are clearly important areas for quality improvement in nursing homes. A gap exists between actual practice and current best practice [47]. Change in this setting is difficult. Nursing homes are already burdened by local, state, and federal policies that regulate licensure and eligibility for reimbursement [39]. Staff turnover is high at many facilities and most of the one-on-one care is provided by nursing aides, many of whom have had little to no formal education [39]. Most patients are followed by physicians who see patients monthly and typically have little role in the management of the facility [39].

There are growing efforts at the state and national level to influence and improve pain management in long-term care. The Joint Commission on the Accreditation of Healthcare Organizations (JCAHO) partnered with the Robert Wood Johnson Foundation to develop a set of pain standards for hospitals, nursing homes, and clinics. The JCAHO Pain Standards went into effect January 1, 2001 and are listed in Table 10.3. These standards emphasize the right of every patient to pain assessment and management, the importance of staff awareness and competency, and the need for adequate patient and staff education. While nursing homes must undergo state licensure and Medicare and Medicaid surveys, JCAHO survey is not required and only about 5% currently submit to this evaluation [39].

Table 10.3 Joint Commission on the Accreditation of Healthcare Organizations (JCAHO) Pain Standards

JCAHO Pain Standards
• Recognize patients' rights to assessment and management of pain
• Assess the nature and intensity of pain in all patients
• Establish safe medication prescription and ordering procedures
• Ensure staff competency and orient new staff in pain assessment and management
• Monitor patients postprocedurely and reassess patient problems appropriately
• Educate patients on the role of pain management in treatment
• Address patients' needs for symptom management in the discharge planning process
• Collect data to monitor performance

Source: Joint Commission on Accreditation of Healthcare Organizations Website (http://www.jcaho.org)

Other efforts and policies may have a more immediate effect on pain assessment in the nursing home setting. The "Pain as a Fifth Vital Sign" concept has been adopted by the Veteran's Administration in an effort to incorporate pain assessment into the routine vital sign measurements for patients. Federal and state legislatures have mandated the adoption of this assessment tool in most states. One such example is the state of California where the following law went into effect on January 1, 2000.

1. It is the intent of the Legislature that pain be assessed and treated promptly, effectively, and for as long as pain persists.
2. Every health facility, licensed pursuant to this chapter shall, as a condition of licensure, include pain as an item to be assessed at the same time as vital signs are taken. The health facility shall insure that pain assessment is performed in a consistent manner that is appropriate to the patient. The pain assessment shall be noted in the patient's chart in a manner consistent with other vital signs.

(Source: The Fifth Vital Sign, Section 1254.7 of the California Health and Safety Code).

Ideally these requirements and other similar policies will help to ensure routine screening for pain in nursing home patients. In addition, policies about the effective use of heating pads, potent analgesic drugs, and the outsourcing of services should be evaluated, as efforts are underway to decrease unnecessary barriers [39].

Conclusion

The identification and treatment of pain comprise an integral component of nursing home care. Over the last 10 years, greater attention has been paid to this under-addressed issue; however, there remains considerable room for improvement. With pressure at the state and local levels along with an increased public interest in pain control, nursing homes will need to continue to make efforts to improve the assessment and management of pain in their patients. Health care providers should cater treatment plans to the special needs of their patients given the limitations of the setting and staff. In general, pain management regimens should be simple and well outlined. They should include long-acting agents when possible to provide longer coverage with fewer doses as well as short-acting medications for pain exacerbations. Special considerations must address potential delays in the medication dosing such as when medications or doses are changed.

Future progress in pain assessment and management in the nursing home requires continued advancement in education, research, and public policy. A recent study on pain management improvement projects in the nursing home found that the adoption of systematic implementation models, clinical decision-making algorithms, an interdisciplinary approach, continuous evaluation of outcomes, and use of on-site resource consultants were effective strategies for addressing this pain in this setting [48]. It is clear that most nurses, nursing aides, and physicians who work in the nursing home setting would benefit from educational programs focused on the special needs of this population and setting. Guidelines for nursing staff on the pain assessment in the cognitively intact and impaired patients are essential for optimal day-to-day pain evaluation and management and important for the accurate completion of the MDS. Further research is needed to expand and improve upon current methods of assessment and treatment. As the nursing home population continues to grow, it is imperative that we are equipped to provide these patients with the premium care that they deserve.

References

1. Besdine RW, Rubenstein LZ, Snyder L. Medical care in the nursing home. Philadelphia: Port City Press; 1996.
2. Kemper P, Murtaugh CM. Lifetime use of nursing home care. N Engl J Med. 1991;324:595–600.
3. Weiner D, Peterson B, Keefe F. Chronic pain-associated behaviors in the nursing home: resident versus caregiver perceptions. Pain. 1999;80:577–88.
4. Ferrell BA. Pain evaluation and management in the nursing home. Ann Intern Med. 1995;123:681–7.
5. Ferrell BA, Ferrell BR, Osterweil D. Pain in the nursing home. J Am Geriatr Soc. 1990;38:409–14.
6. Parmelee PA, Katz IR, Lawton MP. The relation of pain to depression among institutionalized aged. J Gerontol. 1991;46:P15–21.
7. Ferrell BA, Ferrell BR, Rivera L. Pain in cognitively impaired nursing home patients. J Pain Symptom Manage. 1995;10:591–8.
8. Ferrell BA. Pain management in elderly people. J Am Geriatr Soc. 1991;39:64–73.
9. Helme RD, Gibson SJ. Pain in older people. In: Crombie IK, Croft PR, Linton SJ, et al, editors. Epidemiology of pain. Seattle: IASP Press; 1999. p. 103–12.
10. Gibson SJ, Helme RD. Age-related differences in pain perception and report. Clin Geriatr Med. 2001;17:433–56.
11. Roy R, Thomas M. A survey of chronic pain in an elderly population. Can Fam Physician; 1986;32:513–6.
12. Sengstaken EA, King SA. The problems of pain and its detection among geriatric nursing home residents. J Am Geriatr Soc. 1993;41:541–4.
13. Proctor WR, Hirdes JP. Pain and cognitive status among nursing home residents in Canada. Pain Res Manag. 2001;6:119–25.
14. Teno JM, Weitzen S, Wetle R, Mor V. Persistent pain in nursing home residents. JAMA. 2001;285:2081.
15. AGS Panel on Persistent Pain in Older Persons. The management of persistent pain in older persons. J Am Geriatr Soc. 2002;50:S205–24.
16. Cadogan MP, Schnelle JF, Al-Sammarrai NR, et al. A standardized quality assessment system to evaluate pain detection and management in the nursing home. J Am Med Dir Assoc. 2005;6(1):1–9.
17. Cadogan MP, Edelen MO, Lorenz KA, et al. The relationship of reported pain severity to perceived effect on function of nursing home residents. J Gerontol A Biol Sci Med Sci. 2008;63(9):969–73.
18. AGS Panel on the Pharmacological Management of Persistent Pain in Older Persons. Pharmacological management of persistent pain in older persons. J Am Geriatr Soc. 2009;10(6):1062–83.

19. Bernabei R, Gambassi G, Lapane K, et al. Management of pain in elderly patients with cancer. JAMA. 1998;279:1877–82.
20. Fisher SE, Burgio LD, Thorn BE, et al. Pain assessment and management in cognitively impaired nursing home residents: association of certified nursing assistant pain report, Minimum Data Set pain report, and analgesic medication use. J Am Geriatr Soc. 2002;50(1):152–6.
21. Reynolds KS, Hanson LC, DeVellis RF, et al. Disparities in pain management between cognitively intact and cognitively impaired nursing home residents. J Pain Symptom Manage. 2008;35(4):388–96.
22. Engle VF, Graney MJ, Chan A. Accuracy and bias of licensed practical nurse and nursing assistant ratings of nursing home residents' pain. J Gerontol A Biol Sci Med Sci. 2001;56:M405–11.
23. Won AB, Lapane KL, Vallow S, et al. Persistent nonmalignant pain and analgesic prescribing patterns in elderly nursing home residents. J Am Geriatr Soc. 2004;52(6):867–74.
24. Jones KR, Fink RM, Clark L, et al. Nursing home resident barriers to effective pain management: why nursing home residents may not seek pain medication. J Am Med Dir Assoc. 2005;6(1):10–7.
25. Herr KA, Mobily PR. Complexities of pain assessment in the elderly: clinical considerations. J Gerontol Nurs. 1991;17:12–9.
26. Parmelee PA, Smith B, Katz IR. Pain complaints and cognitive status among elderly institution residents. J Am Geriatr Soc. 1993;41:517–22.
27. Morrison RS, Siu AL. A comparison of pain and its treatment in advanced dementia and cognitively intact patients with hip fracture. J Pain Symptom Manage. 2000;19:240–8.
28. Cohen-Mansfield J, Creedon M. Nursing staff members' perceptions of pain indicators in persons with severe dementia. Clin J Pain. 2002;18:64–73.
29. Kovach CR, Griffie J, Muchka S, et al. Nurses' perceptions of pain assessment and treatment in the cognitively impaired elderly. Clin Nurse Spec. 2000;14:215–20.
30. Blumenthal D, Gokhale M, Campbell EG, Weissman JS. Preparedness for clinical practice: reports of graduating residents at academic health centers. JAMA. 2001;286:1027–34.
31. Stein WM, Ferrell BA. Pain management in geriatric fellowship training. Gerontol Geriatr Educ. 1999;20:69–78.
32. Stein WM. Pain in the nursing home. Clin Geriatr Med. 2001;17:575–94.
33. Horgas AL, Dunn K. Pain in nursing home residents. Comparison of residents' self-report and nursing assistants' perceptions. Incongruencies exist in resident and caregiver reports of pain; therefore, pain management education is needed to prevent suffering. J Gerontol Nurs. 2001;27:44–53.
34. Fries BE, Simon SE, Morris JN, Flodstrom C, Bookstein FL. Pain in U.S. nursing homes: validating a pain scale for the minimum data set. Gerontologist. 2001;41:173–9.
35. Krulewitch H, London MR, Skakel VJ, et al. Assessment of pain in cognitively impaired older adults: a comparison of pain assessment tools and their use by nonprofessional caregivers. J Am Geriatr Soc. 2000;48:1607–11.
36. Hurley AC, Volicer BJ, Hanrahan PA, Houde S, Volicer L. Assessment of discomfort in advance Alzheimer patients. Res Nurs Health. 1992;15:369–77.
37. Kovach CR, Noonan PE, Griffie J, et al. The assessment of discomfort in dementia protocol. Pain Manag Nurs. 2002;3:16–27.
38. Hadjistavropoulos T, Herr K, Turk DC, et al. An interdisciplinary expert consensus statement on assessment of pain in older patients. Clin J Pain. 2007;23:S1–43.
39. Ferrell BA. The management of pain in long-term care. Clin J Pain. 2004;20:240–3.
40. Gennari C, Agnusdei D, Camporeale A. Use of calcitonin in the treatment of bone pain associated with osteoporosis. Calcif Tissue Int. 1991;49(Suppl 2):S9–13.
41. Gloth III FM, Gundberg CM, Hollis BW, Haddad JG, Tobin JD. The prevalence of vitamin D deficiency in a cohort of homebound elderly subjects compared to a normative matched population in the United States. JAMA. 1995;274:1683–6.

42. Chapuy MC, Arlot ME, Duboeuf F, et al. Vitamin D3 and calcium to prevent hip fractures in the elderly women. N Engl J Med. 1992;327(23):1637–42.
43. Gloth III FM, Lindsay JM, Zelesnick LB, Greenough III WB. Can vitamin D deficiency produce an unusual pain syndrome? Arch Intern Med. 1991;151:1662–4.
44. Gloth MJ, Matesi AM. Physical therapy and exercise in pain management. Clin Geriatr Med. 2001;17:525–35.
45. Thorsteinsson G. Chronic pain: use of the TENS in the elderly. Geriatrics. 1987;42:75–82.
46. Miller SC, Mor V, Wu N, Gozalo P, Lapane K. Does receipt of hospice care in nursing homes improve the management of pain at the end of life? J Am Geriatr Soc. 2002;50:507–15.
47. Jablonski A, Ersek M. Nursing home staff adherence to evidence-based pain management practices. J Gerontol Nurs. 2009;16:1–7.
48. Swafford KL, Miller LL, Tsai PF, et al. Improving the process of pain care in nursing homes: a literature synthesis. J Am Geriatr Soc. 2009;57(6):1080–7.

Chapter 11
The Politics of Pain: Legislative and Public Policy Issues

F. Michael Gloth, III

> *Just because you do not take an interest in politics doesn't mean politics won't take an interest in you.*
>
> Pericles (430 BC)

Just as it is important to consider the whole patient, it is also important to consider the whole pain challenge. While direct efforts in managing pain are helpful and go a long way in relieving suffering, part of a comprehensive plan must involve indirect care and oversight. Part of this involves politics.

In response to a reporter's comment to a physician running for office for the first time regarding his lack of political experience, a congressman within earshot responded, "He works in the hospital, there's as much politics there as anything I see on the Hill!" In this chapter, the techniques for being more effective in promoting good pain management techniques outside of the realm of direct patient care are covered. Many of the points are illustrated through examples of actual experiences, since the relevant research is not abundant here. This chapter is intended to help all of us be better advocates for pain management and to provide a basis for achieving that goal politically in every venue that might otherwise be an impediment. The politics of pain encompasses far more than that dealing with legislators. It also does not mean that one has to run for Congress, although that is a good place to start...

F.M. Gloth, III (✉)
Division of Geriatric Medicine and Gerontology, Johns Hopkins University
School of Medicine, Baltimore, MD, USA
e-mail: fgloth1@jhmi.edu

F.M. Gloth, III (ed.), *Handbook of Pain Relief in Older Adults: An Evidence-Based Approach*, Aging Medicine, DOI 10.1007/978-1-60761-618-4_11,
© Springer Science+Business Media, LLC 2011

Establishing Representation

In 1998, after becoming frustrated with how health care was being adversely affected by government, and the lack of good leadership and representation in Washington, DC, a young physician in Maryland initiated a campaign for the US Senate, targeting a well-entrenched (and well-funded) incumbent [1]. The odds of actually winning such an election were insurmountable, but the value of such an experience was immeasurable. It provided tremendous insight into what is involved in running for office, and it provided knowledge on the diversity of voters, issues, and public servants. Additionally, it provided valuable contacts and direct interaction with hundreds of political officials and supporters. At the completion of the campaign, two messages were clearly received. First, representation by the health-care profession in government is indeed desperately needed. Health care comprises a substantial portion of governmental budgets at every level. The public seeks greater input from qualified health-care professionals, as do elected officials who recognize the importance of health care and generally acknowledge their own lack of education in this area.

At the beginning of this millenium, one of the most popular Senate Majority leaders in our country's history was a physician [2]. Senator Frist was viewed by the general public, by those who work on Capitol Hill, and by his colleagues in Congress, as bright, caring, and dedicated. This is not the image most people have of politicians, and health-care professionals should recognize and embrace this contrast. Physicians and some other health-care professionals oftentimes have backgrounds that give them an advantage in running a campaign for office. At the outset, the image is a positive one of altruistic advocacy. The health-care profession almost forces one to develop excellent organizational skills. Many physicians, as well as other health-care professionals, have experience in public speaking. This provides a surprising advantage on the campaign circuit. It is astounding how many elected officials are poor public speakers. Simply being able to articulate thoughts in a public forum provides a positive contrast to those who cannot. In many circumstances, the skills associated with leadership and communication, are combined with an intimate knowledge of medicine and at least some direct knowledge of health-care policy as it affects the day-to-day care of patients in a variety of settings. Health-care issues today are often among the top issues of campaigns today, and where they are not, they probably should be.

The world-renowned neurosurgeon, Ben Carson, has always found time to participate in the election process. At a fundraiser at which he was the featured speaker and where one of the candidates in attendance was a physician, he brought to the attention of the audience how important it was to have more physicians serving as representatives in various legislative bodies. He noted that early in our country's history, one could expect about a third of elected representatives in Congress to be physicians. Dr. Carson's home State of Maryland is about to lose the only physician in the State Senate. Fortunately, that same physician (an anesthesiologist), Dr. Andrew Harris, will be headed to Congress in the U.S. House of Representative serving Maryland's First District. In recent elections, physician have been catapulted to leadership positions because of their insight and compassion. The public image of these physician politicians is generally positive, as is the respect on both sides of the political aisle.

For those interested in promoting pain relief, it is much more desirable to have a representative who has first-hand experience and inherently understands the issues of pain management rather than to spend time and effort trying to educate a representative and generate the needed support for the cause. This leads to the next message, which is related to getting that needed representation.

The second message is that simply voting on Election Day is inadequate. The campaigns to increase voter turnout are usually targeted at enclaves that are likely to vote for one party (or, occasionally, one position) or another. It can be argued that the country does not need more voters; it needs more intelligent and discerning voting. The number of people that walk into a voting booth who will vote for issues or candidates unknown to them prior to casting their vote is nothing short of astounding. Too many cannot even name their local representatives. Few have ever met any candidate for whom they will cast a vote. Many will complain about politics and their representatives and even voice strong opinions about needing a change in government. Nonetheless, an incumbent running for reelection will win reelection >90% of the time in the USA [3, 4].

Knowing the Candidates and Having Them Know You

In order to have a real impact on policy and politics, one's personal vote is nowhere near the most important factor. Things that will have a much greater impact involve getting to know the issues and the representatives (see Table 11.1). An insightful person from the health-care profession who can listen and articulate thoughts on subjects will be an invaluable asset to anyone who is involved in making health-care policy. Running for office at any level will provide tremendous insight (and contacts) win or lose. Everyone will not have the time, energy, or resources to take that step, however. There are other ways of getting personal time with elected officials in a supportive environment, and this is also extremely useful (some very successful business people will tell you that it is more useful). Attending a local political Party dinner or similar event where candidates and officials are in attendance provides one of the best ways to

Table 11.1 Tips to health-care professionals for influencing representation

Run for political office (focus on integrity and issues)
Help a promising candidate who is running for political office
Attend smaller political events, especially for candidates early in their careers
Meet with representative (outside of the legislative session when possible)
Write thoughtful, brief letters
Join your professional society(ies)
Understand what is motivating your legislator
Lay the groundwork in advance trying to have support before the vote is taken
Meet a representative's support staff. They often have great influence on issues

interact. Such candidates are anxious to get your vote and your support. Interestingly, local political groups will have fewer participants and much less cost. Candidates realize the importance of gaining the support of such groups, however, and are anxious to curry favor in that setting. Remember, too, that many of these candidates will be in politics for a long time. Eventually, many will be elected officials in positions that have direct or indirect influence on health-care policy or oversight.

Small Contributions Are Appreciated Too

Most people in politics start out with great intentions and are quite personable. In general, they will be genuinely grateful to anyone who has demonstrated any interest and support along the way. Even small contributions at that level are often remembered. Of course, a comment like, "I can remember contributing to your campaign for..." years later will go a long way to jogging that memory.

Contributions do not have to be monetary. Helping during a campaign, especially in smaller contested ones, can be very useful. Participating at the polls at the State Delegate or State Senate level on Election Day will usually be remembered by the candidates, especially if it is a busy professional who takes half of a day off from work to volunteer at a polling place that is likely to have a close vote. If there is little contest in your own election site, then offer to go somewhere where there promises to be a tight race for a promising candidate.

Public officials are inundated by people lobbying (officially and unofficially) for one thing or another. They also must listen to a wide range of constituents. It will be refreshing for them to have a visit with a supporter who is succinct, logical in the presentation of information, and an advocate for someone else, i.e., patients. While visits can be arranged to a representative's office (and are often worthwhile), the timing of such visits should be considered carefully. For many elected officials, there is an "off-season," i.e., that period of time when the legislature is not in session. That is a great time to meet to discuss issues that will require legislation and to work outside the hectic pace of the legislative session.

In Washington, most of your representatives will leave the Capitol on Friday. Hence, this is not the best day to step into their office if you actually want to see them.

For most people that last-minute encounter right before an important vote on the floor will add little beyond stress for your legislator. If they need your input right before the vote, they will find a way to reach you. As an example, one physician who had been actively promoting a piece of legislation related to protections for prescribers of pain medications in the State of Maryland had been told by opposing legislators and lobbyists that the bill would not get out of committee. Once it did, the comments were that it would not get passed on the Floor. The physician was called on his way to a sick patient's home by a key delegate who was about to make his final speech on the topic and wanted to clarify some facts. Later, a call came to the physician from the house floor so that the physician could listen as the final vote fell in favor of the legislation!

As an aside, it is interesting to note that in that particular circumstance, after subsequently passing on the Senate side, the comments to the same physician were that the Governor would veto the legislation and press reports reflected that same sentiment. A major state senator who encountered the physician almost a year later…after the Governor (who was in the same party as this senator which was not the party of the physician) had signed the legislation, was heard to say, "the next time you support a piece of health-care legislation, I hope you'll let me know in advance." The implication was fairly obvious. She had conceded that the piece of legislation was, in the final analysis, a good one. More important was the fact that the physician had played a strategic role in promoting the bill, and that this veteran senator was not only complimenting the physician on adroitly handling the political system but also was looking for an ally in future legislative battles.

Join Your Professional Society

Participating in your professional organization(s) may also be helpful. Simply belonging to the organization will provide opportunities to raise issues that might be embraced by the organization and further developed for ultimate presentation by the organization to legislators or other bodies/individuals that can influence policy. If time constraints prevent active committee participation, do not fret. One can select issues and participate more as matters related to those key issues arise. The other benefit is that such organizations, which have active legislative committees and lobbyists, may promote issues and foster relationships between you and other representatives. This can be helpful, not only for the issue at hand but also for future issues as well. It is also helpful for a representative to know that an interested constituent is active in a large group of potential voters (and contributors).

Resisting Restrictive (and Costly) Regulation and Manipulation

Such involvement in government is also important for health-care professionals because of wide-reaching policy issues. Regulatory oversight of health care has, in many settings, gone awry. Over time, much health-care regulatory oversight has gone from a necessity for keeping vulnerable patients out of harm to a burdensome, punitive system that actually restricts access and may substantially detract from good care for much of the citizenship. Being able to serve as an advocate for patients and facilities that provide good care for patients becomes just one more responsibility that befalls individuals providing clinical care. Knowing regulators, department directors, secretaries of health, etc., either directly or through the person who appointed them to their positions, can also be helpful when the best interest of the patient is the focus.

Politically, pain relief, like hospice, is a great issue. It is hard to argue against it. By assimilation, health-care professionals dealing with pain management will be sought to be advocates for other positions, which may only peripherally include pain management, to move other portions of the legislation ahead. Because of this, there will be many more opportunities to promote pain management issues legislatively and otherwise. This, however, also has a downside. There will be great efforts to manipulate well-intentioned people in the pain field to advocate or oppose legislation, ostensibly on the merits of its proposed impact on pain control efforts. Even a bright group of physicians who would not approve funding for research without an objective assessment of the data may lose some of that usual objectivity and overlook available evidence as proponents or opponents of legislation vie for their attention and support on such issues. It is a danger that may threaten the overall image of pain management advocates, and all would be well advised to be particularly vigilant when multiple issues are at stake.

A classic example evolved as the 106th Congress considered the Pain Relief Promotion Act. Unlike many bills in Congress, this one carried a title that actually reflected at least a part of the intent of the legislation. Paradoxically, some physicians and even some smaller health-related organizations, opposed the legislation, which had specific language to protect the providers who prescribe medications for pain relief, even should such drugs have the potential for untoward events. The wording of the legislation provided protection, even if the medication would increase the risk of death or hasten death in its use to provide pain relief. Few people would argue over the merits of providing pain relief, especially to those individuals with terminal illness who are suffering with pain. However, the legislation also banned physician-assisted suicide. Groups that support physician-assisted suicide, or even euthanasia, found themselves in a quandary. Physician-assisted suicide and certainly euthanasia have not gained widespread support, either in the medical community or in the general public. Seniors, a rapidly growing political force, are particularly leery of measures that may appear to be incremental steps in arbitrarily limiting life. There is, of course, overwhelming support for providing pain relief to those who are suffering. Opposition to the legislation, therefore, could not focus on the assisted suicide component; such forces had to somehow distort the public's perception of the bill [5].

To do this, prominent pain management advocates had to be recruited. The game plan was a familiar one at the time in Washington. The strategy involved deception on a large scale, relying heavily on emotion, with a focused avoidance of the facts. The groups in opposition realized that it was fruitless to try to argue against the merits of a bill that would specifically provide protection for prescribers of pain medication. The tactic would be to convince the public and legislators that somehow the bill would induce exactly the opposite effect.

When someone alleges that the law will be interpreted as meaning exactly the opposite of what it says, warning sirens should go off in one's mind. The premise of the opposition argument was that physicians capable of the highest academic performance through college and then 4 years or more of postgraduate education are somehow incapable of understanding the English language. It also presumes that physicians inundated with regulatory paperwork, in conjunction with excessive patient loads, are, at large, also able to be keenly aware of legislation on Capitol Hill, or elsewhere for that matter.

For this piece of legislation, there were data on how similar legislation performed at the state level. Many states had already passed such legislation. One simply has to examine the impact of such legislation in states where similar bills have been passed. In fact, as is true with much legislation that is proposed in Washington, DC, much of the language had been adapted from Maryland's "Ban on Physician Assisted Suicide" legislation.

In 1999, the debate at the state level was very similar, with even the same "chilling effect" terminology from the opposition. Interestingly, in Maryland, the title of the bill conveyed the more controversial portion of the legislation. Because of a fairly substantial lobbying effort by people who helped craft, and understood, the legislation, key legislators became adequately educated, and a bill that was never supposed to get out of committee, not only passed committee, but also narrowly passed in both the House and the Senate. The politics behind the legislation would prove to be educational for anyone involved in legislative efforts. Maryland, which was essentially a one-party State, passed little, if any legislation that was not viewed as favorable by the Democrats in power. The bill caused a fair amount of rift among the Democrats (interestingly, Republicans were fairly uniform, but did not view this as a party issue). When the bill finally reached the Governor's desk, press releases from the Governor's office immediately went out indicating that the Governor was considering a veto. This made it easy for the Governor to identify the position of a variety of contributors and lobbyists and to get input from his own party (as well as to create some political equity). Ultimately, the Governor signed the legislation and that law had no evidence of a negative effect at all, and certainly no "chilling effect" on pharmaceutical prescribing. In fact, in Maryland, as well as in every state that had such legislation passed, there was an increase in the legitimate prescribing of opioids and other strong medications used for pain control. Indeed, physicians universally expressed a mixture of relief and elation upon knowing that for the first time, such protective legislation existed.

During the discourse with groups opposing the Pain Relief Promotion Act, two things become overtly evident. First, no opposition physician ever cited historical evidence where such legislation had already been enacted. This is because their "chilling effect" had never come to fruition. Second, those individuals who had been well entrenched in movements that have supported either physician-assisted suicide or euthanasia never tried to develop a groundswell, which would have revealed that the real opposition was to a ban on physician-assisted suicide, knowing that such a ban would have made support for euthanasia even less likely. Rather, arguments evolved around physicians' fear of government intervention, that it was a state's rights issue, or that there was concern about involvement of the Drug

Enforcement Agency, all of which were specious arguments that crumbled under close scrutiny of the surrounding facts.

There are many ways to defeat a bill. One can keep it in Committee, one can keep it from a vote on the floor before the session adjourns, or if it makes it to the floor for a vote, it can be voted down. Then, there is always the possibility of a veto from the Executive Branch. There are other less common techniques (e.g., a filibuster) as well. After the session ended without passage of the Pain Relief Promotion Act, one prominent and well-respected physician of the highest integrity and who has done much to promote pain relief (and, incidentally, was receiving funding from an organization that supports the concepts of physician-assisted suicide and euthanasia) stated publicly that one of the primary reasons she voiced opposition to the bill was that it would not have provided enough money to accomplish the goals of pain-relief advocates. Of course, in the final analysis, nothing was appropriated, which makes that argument somewhat apocryphal.

The most important point of the story about the Pain Relief Promotion Act is that many people who are advocates of pain relief found themselves supporting opposite sides. One has to think that experts who opposed the Act either opposed a ban on physician-assisted suicide or were duped. In Maryland, such legislation had little impact on assisted suicide but did help to relieve suffering and ease the burden on health-care professionals who work to provide pain relief. Even the most ardent opposition legislators there have had to concede that the legislation has indeed had a positive impact. It is a lesson for all of us who are going to work to promote pain relief. While there is probably little need (or room) for additional regulatory oversight, we need to be vigilant about what we will support. If legislation is available which is going to foster better pain relief, and there is a desire to oppose the legislation, because of other accompanying baggage, it is important to maintain integrity for future efforts. Many experts lost stature among legislators because those experts took a stand to oppose a bill that supported their basic cause. That loss of trust will hurt as future legislation is considered. It would have been better to oppose the legislation for other reasons or to remain silent on the bill.

The pain management cause is a noble one, and it will gain much more support in the long run if supporters avoid the controversial baggage associated with other issues and resist the temptation to distort or excessively sensationalize the facts to arouse an even stronger emotional response. There are plenty of alarming facts, and the passion for pain relief is high enough for testimony without sensationalism to easily win the day. So, the next time someone expresses concern about the "chilling effect" of a piece of legislation, remember how "chilling" a snow job can be.

Even when genuinely intended to improve pain management, health-care providers, physicians in particular, must be judicious in their assessment of proposed regulations, especially if such regulations are to be legislated. Always ask two questions "Will there be unintended consequences?" and "What are the other motivating factors that may be influencing legislators, or bureaucrats who support legislation and/or new regulations impacting clinician behavior?" Be wary of any legislation or regulation that is put forward and lists "No fiscal impact." P.J. O'Rourke once said, "If you think health care is expensive now, wait until you see what it costs when it's free." Legislation that bears the label "No fiscal impact" generally means that the costs will be paid by private citizens. Oftentimes, those "private citizens" pay the costs as members of affected organizations or businesses. The people who are affected by insurance companies, people who are affected by institutions providing health care, or physicians usually pay the costs of health-care programs that have "no fiscal impact." The cost of health-care legislation or regulation is often measured in lost jobs and increased health-care burden. For example, if everyone has to have a formal pain assessment done every day, then the time and resources necessary to provide that assessment to stable patients without pain will be time and resources that cannot go to patients who have pain and require treatment. In the circumstance of physicians who provide care for seniors, reimbursement has government-mandated caps. This government restriction on wages and salaries to physicians means that physicians can only respond to an increase in regulations by decreasing their earnings and those of their staff or go into another line of work that does not involve such burdensome government restrictions on earnings (wage and price controls).

New regulations and new legislation are almost always costly. If it is directed towards physicians, it will have either direct financial implications, or there will be indirect costs related to documentation, paperwork, and time away from clinical care. Few clinicians envisioned what an onus Medicare would become. The idea that all of us would contribute to Ted Turner's health care after he reaches 65 years of age is a concept that becomes more and more difficult to justify.

The Fear of Legislation Can Be Just as Motivating

It has been said that legislation, like sausage making, is a process that is difficult to watch in its entirety. It should also be recognized that much more is accomplished through the proposal of legislation than through the passage of legislation. Despite the fact that the Clinton Health Plan was generally recognized as being problematic and never passed, many changes took place in health care in preparation for proposed changes. Oftentimes, when legislation that is distasteful passes, it does so because the legislation is filled with "incentives" to purchase support from various groups or from those reluctant to cast a favorable vote. The final legislation on health care that passed in 2010 was one of the more blatant examples of such efforts.

In other arenas, however, the threat of legislative action can provide for desirable changes without any legislation even being introduced. This is nicely illustrated by an example that occurred in Maryland in 2001. In that State, a regulatory agency in the State government was using people who were unqualified to oversee medical care, including pain management practices, in long-term-care facilities. A complaint to the appropriate person in the Department of Health and Mental Hygiene fell on deaf ears.

Now, most bureaucrats in regulatory agencies recognize that a legislative change, i.e., a law, which forces a change within that regulatory agency is one that cannot be altered without additional legislation. This is clearly recognized as a potential loss of power for a bureaucrat, and oftentimes, changes within a regulatory agency can be facilitated simply by the perception that a legislative proposal may result, should action not occur within the agency. Many a bill has been withdrawn before ever being heard by committee, because of ameliorating actions by those potentially most directly affected. As noted previously, it is quite a feat to get a bill with any substantial opposition passed. Despite its intricacies, the legislative process of a Democratic Republic still produces a substantial number of new laws and regulations. Perhaps part of the reason is because the difficult process of passing new legislation is offset by the zeal of legislators and regulators who garner the most attention by passing new regulations, or by proposing new legislation. So, despite all of the obstacles and difficulties, we still probably see more laws passed than are necessary.

With regard to the oversight issue, as soon as a senator in Annapolis proposed legislation to address the issue, the agency director became very accommodating, with assurances that anyone in that oversight position would go through the same type of training that was required of the physicians whose care was being overseen. The newly proposed legislation was never introduced.

Specific Health System Obstacles

Folks who work in the long-term-care environment have recently been confronted with an obstacle to prescribing opioids as well as other Schedule II–V drugs. For years, opioids were prescribed in the same fashion in a nursing home as occurred in the hospital. Interestingly, nurses in the nursing-home setting have not been identified as agents of the physician, as is true in the acute hospital. For this reason, prescribing Schedule II drugs in the nursing home should have actually been very different in the hospital. Common sense ruled the day for years, however, and there was no enforcement of this distinction in the practically similar, but technically different settings. In 2009, a new administration came into power and suddenly the Drug Enforcement Agency (DEA) began to police this practice and levy large fines for noncompliance. Pharmacy providers quickly recognized their liability and policies for prescribing opioids went from accepting a physician order on an order sheet or having nurses take a verbal order for schedule II drugs over the phone to requiring that physicians speak directly with the pharmacist and accompany such discussions with prescriptions regardless of location or time of encounter. In an urgent situation, this requires three separate prescriptions. One must be written for any drug used from an emergency supply kept in the facility, for an immediate dose; a second script for the emergency 3-day supply (the maximum amount that physicians can give by phone); and a third prescription for the regularly dosed schedule II medication that would subsequently be given as routine or as needed.

The DEA was not only adamant about enforcing the law for Schedule II drugs but also extended the practice to Schedule III–V drugs. Despite many discussions with the DEA from multiple specialty organizations and patient advocacy groups, a Congressional hearing was required to develop a more reasonable solution for patients. Unfortunately, as of the time of this chapter's submission, only the most viable solution presented would be acceptable to the DEA, according to Joseph Rannazzisi (the agency's deputy assistant administrator), on whether each state would pass new legislation allowing nursing homes to be registrants like hospitals [6]. Such solutions could assure decades of inadequate pain relief for the most frail and vulnerable portion of our population.

All Politics Are Local

In reality, most of the politics associated with pain management occurs far removed from state or national capitols. Such pain politics flourish in hospitals, with insurance providers, and among colleagues and family members. Beyond good skills in communication and spending time addressing concerns, it is helpful to understand the political dynamics of various settings. Sadly, it is not always as simple as defining what is in the best interest of patients. While many of the principals are indeed similar in the hospital as in a legislative assembly, there are some differences worth addressing.

The Democratic Republic that has served this country so well does not exist within the confines of hospital politics. In some respects, implementing policy changes in a large hospital can be as difficult as passing some laws. Depending on the structure of the hospital, the medical staff may have tremendous impact on whether changes are instituted or not.

Many hospitals have been confronted with the prospect of trying to limit or discourage certain drugs with high adverse event profiles that can easily be substituted with safer drugs that are as, or more, effective. Meperidine has been associated with a host of adverse events in seniors, and it should be avoided in the elderly in particular [7, 8]. Meperidine leads to the formation of a metabolite, normeperidine, which accumulates beyond the analgesic duration of meperidine. Normeperidine acts as a central stimulant, which lowers seizure threshold when used chronically. Additionally, meperidine has been associated with an increased risk of falls, and increased likelihood of sedation and psychotomimetic activity when compared to other opioids [9, 10]. With these facts in mind, many hospitals have taken meperidine off of formulary or restricted its use. Accomplishing such a change is exceedingly difficult in some hospitals. The process involves input from the pharmacy and therapeutics committee. Once a decision is made at that level, members of the administration are notified. Subsequently, the department chairs are notified. Then, the Medical Executive Committee is brought into the decision-making process. If everyone concurs with the decision, the decision is brought to the medical staff. Depending on the influence of the medical staff, there may be sufficient resistance by a few influential (or at least loud) members that the formulary goes unchanged. This is usually done by staff who have not kept up with the literature, but have years of "personal experience." This "personal experience" often amounts to a few anecdotes with no scientific categorization or analysis. An administration that fears retaliation of its medical staff in the form of decreased admission rates is easily manipulated.

On the other hand, a medical staff that acts in the best interest of the patients can be a great asset to the quality of care. It is, in part, because of the symbiotic relationship between hospital physician staff and administration that one can understand why a hospital is no better than its medical staff and the image of the medical staff is quite dependent on the commitment of the administration.

When State Regulators Are Wrong

Oftentimes, those individuals charged with the responsibility of determining when a facility is in violation of regulations or law, themselves lack adequate training and clinical background to make consistently sound judgments. Anyone who has confronted the State over such matters has, in all likelihood, been impressed by the lack of expertise across the table and the arrogance that sometimes is in direct proportion to the level of ignorance. While arrogance and ignorance do a poor marriage make, it is one that is all too common in government officials. Inevitably, if one works in the pain field and in an environment such as the nursing home where the amount of regulation is matched only by that for nuclear power plants and the airline industry, encounters with the State will occur. Some will have reasonable outcomes, but too many will not. Fortunately, there is often recourse by appeal through Federal oversight. Such appeals are often accompanied by a better understanding of the law and regulations, but more importantly less likely to be prejudiced by prior encounters and hearsay. Unfortunately, administrators are often reluctant to pursue appeals due to the fear of retribution in future matters. One recourse to apparently arbitrary and capricious decisions from State regulators would be to have State law or regulations require a greater burden of proof from the State whenever greater penalties are being considered.

Do the Groundwork

As is true with any legislative body, when policy changes are desirable, it is crucial to get as much support as possible BEFORE any presentation to the staff at large is made. Policies should be acceptable to official leadership as well as unofficial but commonly acknowledged leaders in the group. While it should go without saying, all too often basics, like notifying the key players in a policy change before presenting to anyone else, are overlooked. A policy that requires a great deal of nurse approval, should, of course, be presented to the Director of

Nursing at the outset. When spearheading a new program, always distribute credit magnanimously, but be avaricious with blame. One is more likely to get more done that way, and beneficial policy changes are more likely to be successful. In dealing with local policy issues related to pain control, especially for those with national or international reputations who are sought throughout the land for advice, it is advisable to keep this quotation in mind, "A prophet is not without honor except in his native place..." [11] It is always best to address such topics when the local audience is inviting you to do so. Better still, bring in another expert who will have the wherewithal to acknowledge your expertise and invite your comments.

When trying to change policy and garner support, remember, too, that facts are very helpful, but not sufficient alone. Expertise is relevant (and also relative). Everyone will want to have an established and recognized expert on his or her side. Also try to avoid situations that rely on a democratic consensus for all decisions. Unless there is a selection process that has provided appropriate leaders to represent the masses, a pure democracy is doomed to mediocrity.

Lastly, choose committee work carefully. Too many committees lack the funding and power to be truly instrumental in initiating change. Committee work can be time-consuming and unless clearly fruitful in the mission of pain relief may involve time better spent elsewhere.

Helping the Media Help You

Regardless of the setting, part of pain politics must involve the media. Marketing a good idea is as important as the idea itself. Some would argue that it is even more important if the policy or idea is to come into general use. Few would disagree that Beta was better than VHS, that MacIntosh® had a better operating system than Microsoft®. With this in mind, communication is absolutely important. In the local setting, it will be necessary to get involved with local hospital marketing and public relations personnel so that a coherent message introduces a new concept and that there continues to be updates as the policies are introduced. This is true on a larger scale as well. Developing local contacts inevitably leads to larger media contacts. It is always good advice to develop advisory panels for large organizations that deal with pain control or hospice issues. Such advisory panels will want to have leaders in the community, and that should include some helpful members of the media. Such people are likely to embrace such a noble cause as pain relief and help promote the important messages that pertain to it.

When dealing with members of the media, analyze the situation as carefully as examining a wheezing older adult and determining whether the diagnosis is bronchospasm or heart failure. Know whether you will be dealing with print, radio, television, or something else. Recognize that the person doing the interview is doing a job just like anyone else. Answers should be concise and convey the message. Speak slowly enough that the interviewer can type all of the important points and articulate so that there is no question about your message. Be mindful that no reporter is without bias. With pain relief, most are trying to make you sound or appear even better than reality, so the bias works in your favor. However, this is not always the case. Regardless of the tone of the interview, remain courteous and pleasant, but stay on message and always clarify and correct erroneous statements made during the interview. Having said this, being interviewed about promoting pain relief should be a pleasure and anything but hostile. It is acceptable to inform a reporter that you would like to tape the interview as well. This allows you to verify any misquotes and, more importantly, helps you improve, as you review the tape, for next time.

A reporter is looking for something of interest to the reader or listener that can be conveyed in a very short period of time or in a few paragraphs. While you may be interviewed for 20 or 30 min, you are likely to be one of a few people being interviewed and only one or two quotes may appear in the piece. Therefore, emphasize the most important elements of your message, and you may even acknowledge during the interview how important a particular statement is.

For television, a camera crew may be in the office for over an hour for what will be less than a minute of actual airtime. This should emphasize how important it is to be on message every minute of the interview. Some of the most useful time is spent on talk shows with interactions between host and guest or a panel of guests. In such a setting, you will have about 20–40 min (depending on whether the program is in a 30 or 60 min slot). Such programs go quickly, and you may only have time to cover two or three points. It is wise to write down five points that you would like to get across and prioritize them. If at all possible, work to steer the conversation in the direction of some of your key points.

Remember that such programs must constantly search for new topics and new guests. Be gracious and offer to help again some time, should they need someone. Recognize that reporters usually work on a deadline. So, respond as quickly as possible and always leave a way for them to reach you. Try to keep a list of contact phone numbers, fax numbers, and e-mail addresses. This may be useful in providing them with information that relates to pain management when such information is newsworthy.

Always keep in mind other options for getting your message out on the airwaves or in the paper. Talk shows will occasionally discuss pain, or drug abuse, or even a particular drug. Your expertise will be a welcome addition to the show and you are likely to be able to get your message across that way. Remember to enunciate, be brief, and know your message. It always strengthens your message if you do not use space fillers such as "uh," "you know," "um," or "like."

With print media, there are ample opportunities for writing letters to the editor. Expert opinions will almost always get published if an opinion is stated in a clear, concise, and courteous fashion. Do not overlook the electronic print media as well (see Table 11.2). There are many venues for publishing or making a message available. The next chapter deals specifically with the Internet and some options that are likely to be useful in the promotion of pain relief.

Table 11.2 Tips for any health-care professional on using the media to get out the pain message

Send focused and concise letters to the editorCall talk shows when anything related to the topic of pain relief develops

Use group e-mail and faxes to release relevant information to the press in a timely fashion

Get to know reporters and editors (they are good resources for advisory board recruitment)

Stay focused and concise

Do NOT use space fillers (see text)

Challenges from the Media

Finally, recognize that there are some politically correct issues that will have the potential to create havoc even with a topic such as pain relief in older adults. One surrounds the issue of ageism. While racism and sexism is taboo, ageism seems to get a pass in our society. Deprecating remarks about seniors are commonplace, and often they are the brunt of jokes. Rarely does anyone challenge such "humor." People will often target the older population unfairly simply because of age and the stereotypes that accompany aging. It will be important to staunchly defend pain management in seniors and to unmask age bias whenever it is presented.

Another antagonist in pain control discussions is a negative public opinion about the pharmaceutical industry. Some newer and relatively expensive drugs have been demonstrated to be superior to some of the less expensive drugs. There will be tremendous resistance to acknowledging such improvement, since many will interpret such acknowledgement as "advertising." In such circumstances, there is truly a bias; it is a bias against the pharmaceutical industry and the potential for profits. For example, a good academic physician publicly acknowledged that a particular nonsteroidal anti-inflammatory drug, classified as a COX-2 specific agent, is safer for the gastrointestinal tract than a traditional nonsteroidal anti-inflammatory drug. However, because of a bias against any data from any study involving funding from the pharmaceutical industry, there are some physicians who refuse to be swayed by the plethora of data and the US Food and Drug Administration's acknowledgment of increased safety and would not write for such a drug [12]. In essence, there was a willingness to chance putting an elderly patient at increased risk for intestinal bleeding, because of the increased short-term cost of the safer medication and a bias against industry. When the American Geriatrics Society (AGS) published guidelines on the Management of Persistent Pain in Older Adults, the committee members who authored them were accused by a few members of the AGS of being unduly influenced by big drug companies [13]. As this illustrates, if even well-educated physicians are unduly affected by preconception, dealing with an uneducated public can be a daunting challenge. Whenever integrity warrants doing what is right, even when politically difficult, everyone would be wise to remember the advice of a pilot who remarked, "When the flak is heaviest, you're usually right over the target."

A few reports of OxyContin abuse in rural Virginia left a perfect opportunity for the media to create a story and run with it. It got to be so absurd that the media's distortion of reality (the media hype almost certainly led to far more abuse of this medication than would have ever occurred without the sensational press reports) itself became newsworthy [14].

The tragedy of such irresponsible "journalism" of course is the devastating consequences to members of our society. This venture, beyond covering a problem to *causing* one, by advertising to abusers the existence of a new drug, and how to get and use it, forces health-care professionals to divert valuable resources trying to get accurate information to the public at-large and patients, in particular. Perhaps worse, the media-propagated panic makes doctors and legitimate users needlessly afraid of utilizing an important advance in the treatment of pain. It also damages the efforts to positively educate the public about the merits of such medications.

This same problem develops when advertisements from malpractice attorneys hopeful in getting out-of-court settlements advertise to acquire any patient who has had the misfortune of having a medical problem while taking a medication. Opportunistic attorneys who will then advertise state to state to recruit such patients also, often, produce great anxiety among patients taking medications that are needed for controlling pain and other symptoms or risk factors. In an open society where free speech is the hallmark of our freedom, the recourse is limited. Regardless of one's stand on such issues, it would be easy to debate the frequently high harm to benefit ratio that hurts patients and requires a diversion of valuable time and energy from health-care professionals directing pain control efforts.

To be most successful in managing pain, physicians and other health-care professionals cannot be content with direct patient care alone. It is useful and necessary to place the "political" and "social" aspects of pain relief on the professional calendar because it constantly plays into how we practice medicine and how successfully we manage pain.

Conclusion

In summary, beyond efforts directed toward our patients, our efforts to provide pain relief for seniors must be broader, with attention to legislative and health-policy issues. A part of the solution for pain involves indirect care and oversight. Part of this involves politics. By this, it must be understood that it is more than identifying political leaders who are likely to be supportive of pain relief as a noble cause (although that does make up a small part of the politics of pain). There is actually much, much more, and it is also not just related to Federal or State government. The politics of pain must be addressed locally, in the hospitals, with advocacy groups, with colleagues, with family members, with third party payers, and with the media. Encouraging everyone to take a strong interest and participate in the legislative process is, of course, also part of the solution to poor pain management. It needs to be clear, however, that the solution to pain management does not lie solely in regulation or legislation. From requirements of Institutional Review Boards to reimbursement-related documentation, pressures have been placed on paperwork in deference to protecting patients from pain. We cannot mandate our way to good pain control. There must be improved education and advocacy at every level. Everyone must recognize the ability to obtain pain relief and work to assure that everyone receives it. Allowing pain to persist is an injustice and as has often been said, "An injustice to one is an injustice to all!"

Tips for Overcoming Policy and System Barriers

Get involved...even run for office...you are better qualified than you may think

Support some candidates running for office both with time commitments and money

Join your professional society and become active

Know your representatives (and importantly be sure that they know you)

Pursue other avenues and do not get discouraged

Be polite and respectful

References

1. LaDuc D. Physician Seeks GOP Nomination to Face Mikulski. Washington Post, March 24, 1998; A16.
2. First Elected GOP Senate Leader. Washington Times. December 24, 2002: A1. Article ID: 200212240851380021.
3. Greenberg D. Term limits the only way to clean up Congress 2003. http://www.heritage.org/Research/GovernmentReform/BG994.cfm. Available at time of publication 2003.
4. Ornstein NJ, Mann TE, Malbin MJ. Vital Statistics on Congress 1993–1994. Washington, DC: American Enterprise Institute for Public Policy Research; 1994. p. 118, table 4–7.
5. Gloth III, FM. Chilling effect or just a snow job? 2003. http://www.seniorhealthcare.org/Srhealth.nsf/pubPOLframe!OpenPage under "Commentary". Available at the time of publication 2003.
6. Haglund K. Senate Committee Probes DEA actions. Caring for the Ages. 2010;11:19.
7. Stein WM. Cancer pain in the elderly. In: Ferrell BR, Ferrell BA, editors. Pain in the elderly. Seattle: IASP Press; 1996. p. 69–80.
8. Beers MH. Explicit criteria for determining potentially inappropriate medication use by the elderly. Arch Intern Med. 1997;157:1531–36.
9. Marcantonio ER, Juarez G, Goldman L, Mangione CM, Ludwig LE, Lind L, et al. The relationship of post-operative delirium with psychoactive medications. JAMA. 1994; 27219:1518.
10. Shorr RI, Griffin MR, Daugherty JR, Ray WA. Opioid analgesics & risk of hip fracture. J Gerontol. 1992;47:M111–5.
11. Christ J. The Bible. Mark 6:4.
12. U.S. Food and Drug Administration. FDA approves new indication and label changes for arthritis drug, VIOXX. FDA Talk Paper. 2002. http://www.fda.gov/bbs/topics/ANSWERS/2002/ANS01145.html. 11 Apr 2002.
13. The AGS Panel on Persistent Pain in Older Persons. The management of persistent pain in older adults. J Am Geriatr Soc. 2002;50(Suppl 6):S205–24.
14. Kaushik S. OxyCon Job: the media-made Oxycontin drug scare. The Cleveland Free Times. May 7, 2001 Cover Story.

Chapter 12
The Internet and Electronic Medical Records to Assist with Pain Relief

F. Michael Gloth, III

> *You can be on the pulse of medicine or just checking to see if there still is one.*

Patty Gloth

The use of computers and the internet to improve information and communication as a conduit for improving pain control was discussed in the first edition of the *Handbook of Pain Relief in Older Adults*. Since that time, there have been few changes that have standardized electronic health records to allow for adequate handling of pain issues. The literature continues to be devoid of meaningful discussions on this issue as well. Nonetheless, computer technology provides a tremendous opportunity to improve the overall care of patients, particularly those in pain. This chapter comments on the use of the internet and electronic medical record (EMR) systems to facilitate improved pain management.

People who work in the pain management field are quick to acknowledge that few patients with chronic pain have not explored most available resources on pain control and many have experimented with alternative therapies in hopes of finding pain relief. The internet has offered greater access to information but has also made it difficult to discern between what information is based on medical science and what is apocryphal. Even health-care professionals have some difficulty identifying reputable web sites for pain management. Because the public relies on the physician or other primary-care provider for medical care, it stands to reason that the best source for reliable medical information is that same person. Regarding pain, studies indicate that health-care providers often lack knowledge about pain management [1, 2]. This makes choosing a worthwhile web site for such information more difficult. This chapter gives some guidance on web site selection and provides some additional guidance on how EMR (sometimes called computerized

F.M. Gloth, III (✉)
Division of Geriatric Medicine and Gerontology, Johns Hopkins University
School of Medicine, Baltimore, MD, USA
e-mail: fgloth1@jhmi.edu

F.M. Gloth, III (ed.), *Handbook of Pain Relief in Older Adults: An Evidence-Based Approach*, Aging Medicine, DOI 10.1007/978-1-60761-618-4_12,
© Springer Science+Business Media, LLC 2011

patient records or CPR, but CPR is too anxiety provoking in the medical profession so here "EMR" will be used!) can also improve treatment plans, especially when the clinician does not have a strong background in pain management.

Seniors and the Internet

Seniors are quite health conscious and, with a third of their income going to health-related expenditures, it is easy to understand why. Census data indicate that in 2009 over 40% of adults 65 years of age or older used computers and the internet [3]. Compare this to estimates that only about 16% of the population over 65 years of age, were using computers in 2000 and, as of 1997, <10% of people over the age of 55 were using the internet [4].

The numbers seem to be increasing both because older adults are learning to use computers and because younger individuals who have relied on computers for business, etc., are aging with those skills in place. It is estimated that, of those seniors who do own a computer in the USA, almost all surf the Web [3]. Even with these encouraging numbers in mind, the reality is that the job of online information finding for many seniors often resides with their children who are voracious users of the internet and computers. Physician use of computers and the internet is understandably high as well. The potential for information sharing on the World Wide Web and the opportunity for EMR to positively impact medical information accumulation and exchange is obvious but also very exciting. Additionally, the current technology presents unusual opportunities for bringing experts from around the globe to the most remote regions of the world in a consultative fashion without ever leaving the home office.

EMR Use

Despite the obvious benefits to EMR, currently less than 10% of physicians use EMR in their practices [5, 6]. Many forces are working to move physicians in the EMR direction, and it might not surprise many people if, in 10 years, only 10% of physicians will not be using EMR. It will enhance care and revolutionize the practice of medicine, particularly as it relates to pain relief. As people scramble to enhance security and assure privacy of patient records, more and more awareness of the advantages that EMR offer will accelerate this transition phase for physicians.

Communication between physician and patient becomes even more important in seniors when trying to achieve adequate pain control. Given the higher prevalence of functional disability in seniors and the recognition that, as the baby boomers age, computer use will be more prevalent, it only makes sense to try to use this technology to enhance communication and the transfer of useful information in an attempt to improve patient care, in particular, pain relief [7]. Computers and the internet will also provide new venues for collecting data in the course of clinical trials and will assist with quality assurance/improvement efforts.

Internet Sites of Interest

First, let us address internet sites that are available for information on pain management. There are many, and it makes sense to divide them into the following categories: advocacy sites for patients in pain, sites to help locate a pain specialist, and sites that provide direct pain management guidance. There will be some overlap but this is a good start. Each site was personally reviewed one final time right before publication and a brief description appears after each web site listing.

Pain Advocacy Web Sites

http://adultpain.nursing.uiowa.edu/ An informational site intended to educate health professionals, patients, and families.

http://www.geriatricpain.org/Pages/home.aspx The purpose of this web resource (GeriatricPain.org) is to identify and share best practice tools and resources that support recommendations for good pain assessment and management in older adults. The web site is organized into categories of emphasis with tools selected to assist nurses with responsibility for pain care in the nursing home.

http://www.jcaho.org This is the website for the Joint Commission on Accreditation of Health Care Organizations (JCAHO) and was established in a joint effort with the University of Wisconsin Medical School, which has done a great deal of work to improve pain management.

http://www.medsch.wisc.edu/painpolicy/ The Pain & Policy Studies Group facilitates public access to information about pain relief and public policy. The Pain & Policy Studies Group, at the University of Wisconsin, addresses both domestic and international policy issues and is a World Health Organization Collaborating Center for Policy and Communications in Cancer Care.

http://www.paincare.org The National Foundation for the Treatment of Pain (through the American Academy of Pain Medicine). This organization is dedicated to providing support for patients who are suffering from intractable pain, their families, friends, and the physicians who treat them.

http://www.painfoundation.org This web site was created by the American Pain Foundation, a somewhat political organization funded by George Soros as an advocacy group primarily focused on relieving pain.

http://www.partnersagainstpain.com This web site is run by Purdue Pharma, Inc. which is a pharmaceutical company that manufactures many analgesics and pain-related medications. It does have a large number of resources and a broad body of information on pain relief for professional and public audiences.

http://www.theacpa.org This site was developed by the American Chronic Pain Association. This organization offers support and information for patients with chronic pain, their families, and support groups.

Pain Web Sites That Help to Identify Specialists in Pain Management

http://www.aapainmanage.org This website, which was developed by the American Academy of Pain Management, has a searchable database of medical facilities that have passed the American Academy of Pain Management's Pain Program Accreditation testing and on-site inspection. This site is not recommended if searching for a geriatrician with pain expertise.

Pain Web Sites That Provide Pain Management Guidance

http://www.guideline.gov This website is a government-run site that catalogs guidelines in many areas. Of over 825 guidelines that are indexed, over 200 are related to pain management. While some are to seniors, a search as of May 2010 failed to list the American Geriatrics Society's guidelines on chronic or persistent pain from 1998, 2002, or 2009.

http://www.painmed.org This website was developed in partnership by the American Academy of Pain Medicine (AAPM) and the American Pain Society (APS). It provides an impartial, consensus on "The Use of Opioids for the Treatment of Chronic Pain," "The Necessity for Early Evaluation and Treatment of the Chronic Pain Patient" and "End of Life." It was designed to address inquiries from state legislatures, medical examiners, regulators, and doctors regarding the appropriate use of opioids among other issues.

http://www.ampainsoc.org This is the website of the American Pain Society and provides guidelines on pain management, information on upcoming meetings and events, as well as position statements.

http://www.stoppain.org The Department of Pain Medicine and Palliative Care at Beth Israel Medical Center runs this site, which is dedicated to providing comprehensive care of the highest quality in pain management and palliative care, and advancing the educational and research aims of these disciplines.

http://www.seniorhealthcare.org This website has both a public and professional side. It includes articles, an "ask the expert" page, and presentation slides for downloading, as well as sections on resources and public policy.

http://www.nlm.nih.gov/medlineplus/pain.html National Library of Medicine/ National Institutes of Health (NLM/NIH) Resources on Pain Links to resources from the National Institutes of Health, the American Geriatrics Society, the Mayo Foundation for Medical Education and Research, the American Society of Anesthesiologists, and more.

http://www.sppm.org This is the website for the Society for Pain Practice Management (SPPM). There is information on upcoming SPPM meetings, on pain syndromes, on the diagnosis and treatment of pain, on new pain management codes, on new developments related to billing and legislation, and on disability insurance. There is also a directory where everyone can place information about their pain practice.

http://www.ninds.nih.gov/health_and_medical/pubs/chronic_pain_htr.htm This publication of the National Institute of Neurological Disorders and Stroke, designed for patients, outlines theories of pain and discusses treatments.

Web Sites That Rate Internet Sites

http://www.painandhealth.org This site is maintained by the Mayday Pain Project. It provides screened lists of internet resources. These lists address such subjects as arthritis pain, cancer pain, fibromyalgia, headache pain, and occupational pain. In addition, separate areas of the site cover pharmacology, pain and rehabilitation, hospitals and therapy, and general pain. Other areas focus on senior pain and pediatric pain. As of 2003, the senior pain internet sites had not been updated for years, which explains the absence of some of the better senior pain web sites. Links may produce some unwanted advertising.

Other Web Sites

http://www.americangeriatrics.org/health_care_professionals/clinical_practice/ clinical_guidelines_recommendations/persistent_pain_executive_summary The American Geriatrics Society has provided this site that includes the Guidelines for Management of Persistent Pain in Older Adults. The executive summary of the guidelines is available now, and readers may view the summary at this website.

http://www.iasp-pain.org This is the website for the International Association for the Study of Pain. The site provides information about continuing education, IASP grants and publications, meetings, and job opportunities.

http://www.aahpm.org This is the site of the American Academy of Hospice and Palliative Medicine (AAHPM). This is a fairly rudimentary site with much of the information out of date. For example, as of 2003, the page entitled "Recent Articles of Interest" had not been updated since January of 1999.

http://www.druglibrary.org/schaffer/asap This site was created by the American Society for Action on Pain, an organization developed by an unrelieved pain victim. The organization deals with public policy relative to pain management and opioids. The site has an array of articles and guidelines including the California Board of Registered Nurses "Pain management policy," "Opioid pain killers available in the USA," and "The Tragedy of Needless Pain."

Web Sites on Diseases Where Pain Is the Predominant Feature

Fibromyalgia

http://www.fmaa.org/ Fibromyalgia Alliance of America (FMAA). Source for information on fibromyalgia, including lists of health-care professionals and support groups specializing in fibromyalgia. The site is in the process of being expanded.

http://www.afsafund.org American Fibromyalgia Association, Inc.

Arthritis

http://www.arthritis.org Arthritis Foundation.

http://www.hopkins-arthritis.com Hopkins Arthritis Center CME, case reports, meeting highlights, "Hear the lecture series," "The role of opioids for chronic pain," and more. Sign up to have news updates delivered to your email.

Headache

http://www.ahsnet.org The American Headache Society [AHS] (formerly known as the American Association for the Study of Headache [AASH]) and the American Council for Headache Education (www.achenet.org), AHS is for health-care professionals and ACHE for patients. The AHS site offers CME, headache information, cassettes of scientific meetings, and instructions on how to subscribe to the journal *Headache* and how to join the Society.

Migraine

http://www.migraines.org M.A.G.N.U.M. The National Migraine Association.

Neuropathic Pain

http://www.sfn.org/briefings/neuropathic.html Neuropathic Pain – A "BrainBriefing" from the Society for Neuroscience: This article describes several promising agents being developed to provide pain-controlling therapies for patients with neuropathic pain, "which results from a nervous system malfunction set off by nerve damage from diseases such as diabetes, trauma, or toxic doses of drugs."

Sickle Cell Disease

http://www.sicklecelldisease.org Sickle Cell Disease Association of America, Inc. oversees this site which is updated on a regular basis.

Pelvic Pain

http://www.pelvicpain.org/ The International Pelvic Pain Society runs this site. Find a calendar of events, membership information, a patient booklet, and copies of the Society newsletter. According to the site, the Society "was incorporated to allow physicians, psychologists, physical therapists and basic scientists to coordinate, collect, and apply" the therapies available for the millions of women with chronic pelvic pain.

Vulvar Pain

http://www.vulvarpainfoundation.org Vulvar Pain Foundation.

Head and Neck Pain

http://www.aahnfp.org American Academy of Head, Neck and Facial Pain developed this site for health-care professionals, including dental professionals: a source of information on products and educational materials, and more. For the public: "a quick and easy way to locate Medical and Dental Professional Members in your area who have specialized knowledge and skills" in the field of head, neck, and facial pain.

EMR to Improve Pain Relief

One would not evaluate the heart in the same way as Sir William Osler in the 1800s, but, curiously, most physicians still keep their medical records the same way. While the medical profession has embraced the advances in technology for most aspects of medicine, including 3D echocardiography, magnetic resonance imaging, and polymerase chain reactions, there has been a tremendous reluctance to embrace a computerized version of the electronic medical record. The reasons are somewhat puzzling, since the billing side of medicine has gone almost completely electronic.

The enigma persists after evaluating the potential improvements in patient care and in cost-effectiveness. For example, EMR facilitates acquisition of information and can reduce adverse events [8, 9]. The benefit is particularly attractive when dealing with frail seniors in pain. A good EMR can also provide treatment recommendations, which can foster improved pain management without the punitive intrusion of government-mandated regulations nor the inconvenience and annoyance of formularies and prior authorization requirements [10, 11]. This concept of improved compliance with clinical recommendations and guidelines should be associated with reductions in medical error rates [12, 13]. Even basic advantages become obvious. For example, EMR systems can instantly resolve issues associated with poor handwriting. By providing electronic prescriptions directly to the pharmacy, not only are transcription errors or misunderstood verbal communications eliminated, the opportunity for alterations and drug diversions are drastically reduced. Medical note writing is streamlined and communication of medical information improves [14]. Some EMR packages will produce automated patient or referral letters based on diagnoses. EMR programs represent a more efficient system, which would allow more time with patients, something health-care providers want as much as patients.

Cost savings occur as well. EMR can reduce the cost associated with dictation, transcription, and medical record storage space requirements (and costs) [15, 16]. Since record retrieval is easier, there is more time for personnel to direct efforts in a more productive fashion. The potential advantage for quality assurance and research can easily be envisioned as well. Chart auditing can even be done remotely. The potential for saving time and effort on this tedious process makes a web-based product very attractive. Role-specific authorization also can increase privacy. Consider that old paper charts are essentially accessible to anyone in the office. With an EMR system, front office staff could quite conceivably no longer have access to personal elements of a medical history. Rather, access could easily be restricted to the demographic information or whatever elements are necessary to fulfill the job role in the office.

In reviewing an EMR system one should identify a system that fulfills the needs of the individual practice model. Large confined hospital systems may be able to depend on a less flexible system. A private office system must be able to cross a variety of health-care systems and settings and cannot be too costly. Systems can go from as little as a few thousand dollars to six figure systems. Table 12.1 gives some features that may appeal to the majority of providers and some factors that will help decide which system is the best fit for any particular practice environment.

Charles Safran at Harvard Medical School once stated, "The promise of electronic patient records is real and proven, but the reality for physicians in the USA has been largely unrealized" [17]. As we struggle with reimbursement issues for pain visits, the improved efficiency and billing opportunities from EMR offer financial survival in addition to the merits of improved patient care [18]. EMR systems also potentially can facilitate regulatory compliance and minimize associated redundancies in the documentation required in the administration of medical care,

Table 12.1 Questions for a practice prior to purchasing an EMR package

1. Is the system accessible offsite? – Ideally, a web-based system with no excess hardware or software costs, no IT personnel requirements, and no need to transfer information between machines or offices is most desirable. Multiple physicians can have access to multiple sites when authorized. More sophisticated systems even allow consultants to have temporary access to needed records

2. Is there template variability and flexibility? – A system that can adapt to individual preferences and can be modified on a large-scale rapidly as medical knowledge advances is most desirable

3. Is there excessive use of menus and templates? – Some systems are so template and algorithm dependent that it will take excessive time to write routine notes. Ideally, a system will incorporate rich text fields with templates to allow for optimally efficient information entry and provide smoother transitions for future notes

4. Is there treatment and prescription automation? – Simply choosing a diagnosis should be followed by automated prescriptions and treatment plans. Most desirable is a system that "learns" from prior input

5. Does the system allow for personal and specialty adaptation? – Individuals should be able to easily modify templates and treatment protocols to accommodate specialty or personal preferences

6. Is there web-reference accessibility while working in a patient record? – Web site availability for assistance based on personal preferences without leaving the medical record should be part of the standard package

7. Does the EMR provide automated calculations and trend graphing for ease in following clinically relevant changes? – This helps identify problems and changes that may anticipate problems

8. Does the system have automated E&M coding? – By calculating the bill in an automated fashion reimbursement improves (with less "undercoding") and there is less chance of inadvertent fraud

9. Is there secure access? – Only a few EMR packages can provide increased ease of Health Insurance Portability and Accountability Act (HIPAA) compliance and role-specific access/authorization. This assures a more secure environment than hard copy records currently in use

10. Does the system provide for integration into other data systems? –Reductions in prescription and other medical errors should be inherent. Physician handwriting no longer comes into play. Coordination with laboratory databases should allow for direct entry into the medical record

11. Does this system actually reduce space requirements? – Some systems require so much additional equipment and storage to update so that the benefit of file space savings is almost lost

12. Is the system sufficiently automated to also reduce transcription costs? – While most voice-activated systems leave much to be desired, the technology will get to a point that it will be quite beneficial. In such circumstances one should have a system that will blend well with voice activation systems. Additionally, the system should have sufficient use of templates and flexibility in modifying templates and to be able to download information from prior records in such a fashion that verbal dictation is essentially eliminated

13. Is the system capable of doing rapid searches of information? – Such systems should be able to improved quality assurance and improve research potential. Rapid analyses of guideline compliance and patient screening should be available

(continued)

Table 12.1 (continued)

14. Is the system capable of downloading old record information and modifying templates without leaving a patient record? – Too many systems require outdated "cut and paste" techniques. Some even require leaving a record to make changes or to obtain prior information. This wastes time and the inefficiency is too tedious

15. Is there capability for secure patient access or authorized family member access? – This can help reduce requests for patient records, help to keep caregivers abreast of medical regimen changes, and save staff time for acquiring and copying records for patients

an issue quite prominent in long-term care. This assistance may help to assuage physicians from fleeing care for seniors [19].

Overall EMR offers the opportunity for better care for patients in pain and it can come with a smaller price tag. Physicians are starting to use the internet to educate patient populations and health-care professionals. The technology exists for modifying the most rudimentary elements of patient care to the benefit of the masses. Unless one believes that the future of medicine will involve less documentation, less redundancy, less bureaucracy, and less government intervention, or unless retirement is in the near future, EMR is a necessary investment.

Conclusion

Our generation is experiencing changes in data collection and retrieval and in communicating such information. The technological advantages stand to revolutionize the practice of medicine.

References

1. Von Roenn JH, Cleeland CS, Gonin R, et al[AU2]. Physician attitudes and practice in cancer pain management. A survey from the Eastern Cooperative Oncology Group. Ann Intern Med. 1993;119:121–6.
2. Hitchcock LS, Ferrell BR, McCaffery M. The experience of chronic nonmalignant pain. J Pain Symptom Manage. 1994;9:312–8.
3. US Census Bureau. Adult computer and adult internet users by selected characteristics: 2000 to 2009. 2010. http://www.census.gov/compendia/statab/2010/tables/10s1121.pdf. Accessed 30 April 2010.
4. Online source from 2003 at time of publication. http://www.accurateonline.com/promotion-articles/internet-stats.htm
5. Maguire P. For doctors, the pressure is on to computerize. ACP-ASIM Observer. 2002;22:1.
6. DesRoches CM, Campbell EG, Rao SR, et al. Electronic health records in ambulatory care – a national survey of physicians. N Engl J Med. 2008;359:50–60.
7. Freedman VA, Martin LG, Schoeni RF. Recent trends in disability and functioning among older adults in the United States: a systematic review. JAMA. 2002;288:3137–46.
8. Keeler J. No more paper. Advance for Health Information Executives. 2001;51–4.

9. Drazen E, Killbridge P, Metzger J, Turisco F. A primer on physician order entry. California Healthcare Foundation. 1 September 2000;1–44.

10. Gloth FM III. Electronic medical record systems: "high tech" helps foster "high-touch" medicine. The Medical Bulletin. 2002;4(10):2.

11. Torppey M. Demonstration on Victory Springs Smart E-Records™. American College of Physicians Maryland chapter meeting, 2003. Available from: http://www.victorysprings.com.

12. Morris AH. Decision support and safety of clinical environments. Qual Saf Health Care. 2002;11:69–75.

13. Kohn LT, Corrigan JM, Donaldson MS, editors. Committee on Quality of Health Care In America. To err is human: building a safer health system. Washington: Institute of Medicine, National Academy; 2000.

14. Safran C, Rind DM, Davis RB, et al. Guidelines for the management of HIV infection in a computer-based medical record. Lancet. 195;246:341–6.

15. Moore PL. Does your EMR=ROI? Physicians Practice. 2002; May/June: 51–4.

16. Gloth III FM, Torppey M. Electronic medical records in clinical care: using "high tech" for "high touch" medicine. American Academy of Hospice and Palliative Medicine Annual Meeting Program. 2003; Abstract no. 601.

17. Safran C. Electronic medical records: a decade of experience. JAMA. 2001;285:1766.

18. Safran C, Sands DZ, Rind DM. Online medical records: a decade of experience. Methods Inf Med. 1999;38:308–12.

19. Pear R. Many doctors shun patients with Medicare. New York Times. 17March 2002; Final Section, Late edition, page 1, Col 5.

Chapter 13
Navigating Pain Care: Trials, Tribulations, and Triumphs and Resources to Help

Micke Brown and Amanda Crowe

> *One person can make a difference and every person must try.*
>
> John F Kennedy

> *If we know that pain and suffering can be alleviated and we do nothing about it, we, ourselves, are tormentors.*
>
> Primo Levi, Concentration Camp Survivor, Chemist, Philosopher

> *Hope is like a road in the country: there was never a road, but when many people walk on it, the road comes into existence.*
>
> Lin Yutang

Pain does not discriminate. It affects people of all races, economic status, and life stages – from our very young to our elders. While pain is common among older adults, it tends not to be adequately treated or managed.

Sadly, many patients live behind a veil of anguish for months – even years – before seeking or finding effective treatment for their pain. There are many reasons for this. One particular challenge is that our society holds stoicism as the preferred norm for acceptable behavior. That is, many think that personal struggles, such as pain, should remain undisclosed or kept a secret – not unlike mental illness or addictive disease.

Our elders may also incorrectly assume that pain is a normal part of aging, or perhaps they do not want to be perceived as complainers, or burdens to their loved ones [1]. They may also delay seeking medical attention because they are concerned about the additional inconvenience or economic hardship that increased diagnostic testing or additional medications may cause. The fear that the provision

M. Brown (✉)
Communications Director, American Pain Foundation
e-mail: mbrown@painfoundation.org

F.M. Gloth, III (ed.), *Handbook of Pain Relief in Older Adults: An Evidence-Based Approach*, Aging Medicine, DOI 10.1007/978-1-60761-618-4_13,
© Springer Science+Business Media, LLC 2011

of adequate pain care may distract their health-care provider from treating a primary, life-threatening illness such as cancer or heart disease has also been reported.

Older patients, in particular, may be hesitant to question the authority of their medical professional and may not persist in seeking the pain treatment they need. For the most part, older generations have not yet accepted the new consumer-driven, patient-centered model of care in which individuals play a more active role in health-care decisions. Unlike younger generations, they may not educate themselves or be as assertive or inquisitive about the care they receive. It is anticipated that as the baby-boom generation continues to age, the prevailing style of "patient-provider" communication will shift toward consumer centricity.

Moreover, older adults frequently live with multiple medical conditions that require ongoing care and treatment. Depending on their insurance coverage or geographic location, patients may not have access to specialists in pain management or geriatrics. In our work with the American Pain Foundation (APF), we hear countless stories about how pain robs people of their livelihood and sense of self. Consider the following letter received by APF in 2009:

Dear APF:

Sadly, I wanted to tell you that my 82-year-old father, a WWII Vet, was forced to suddenly spend two weeks without his pain medication… He had been on it for five years as he underwent treatment for prostate cancer. A new doctor became his physician after his former one retired and refused to continue prescribing the medication fearful that he was either misusing or diverting as he had asked for an early refill. He abruptly stopped the medicine that helped relieve his pain and allowed him to live independently. I watched helplessly as my Dad went through withdrawal with not help from his medical team. It forced him back to the hospital. He died a week later due to a massive stroke. I cannot help but blame his new doctor for causing his untimely death. That will haunt me the rest of my life. Please keep up the work fighting this mindset that pain medication is evil. I have breast cancer, am a nurse practitioner and too weak to do much more.

A common thread among these personal accounts is the uphill battle many people face when trying to find a health-care provider who is willing to treat their pain condition *and* has the requisite skills and training in pain management.

It is critical that practitioners understand the barriers to quality pain assessment and treatment among older patients. The undertreatment of pain is only expected to become more problematic as the baby-boomer population ages and life expectancy increases. The good news is that older people with pain can be effectively treated and, in turn, pain-related morbidity – and even premature mortality – can and should be obviated.

In this chapter, we briefly review some of the challenges to effective pain management in older adults and the importance of empowering them to advocate for their own care, including self-care tips to share with patients and their families and a list of helpful resources.

Challenges Aplenty

With rare exception, everyone experiences pain at some point – a pounding head-ache at the end of a long day, a throbbing toothache warning of a cavity or infection, an open wound or a sprained ankle from a fall, or a stinging burn from touching a hot pan. Pain is the body's natural alarm system, alerting us that something is not quite right. But, when pain persists beyond the point of healing, it can wreak havoc on a person's physical, emotional, and spiritual well-being. Unfortunately, chronic pain is often inadequately assessed and treated, resulting in needless suffering and poor patient outcomes.

Whether it is from an old injury, bone or joint disorders, or other chronic illnesses such as cancer, heart disease, or diabetes, chronic pain in older adults can be challenging to manage. In addition to the challenges mentioned earlier, consider the following:

Common Pain Conditions in Older Adults

- Arthritis.
- Lower back and neck pain; vertebral compression fractures from osteoporosis.
- Abdominal pain (e.g., gallstones, bowel obstruction, peptic ulcer disease, abdominal aortic aneurysm).
- Cancer-related pain (symptom of disease or effect of nerve damage from treatments).
- Neuropathic pain due to diabetes, herpes zoster ("shingles"), kidney disease, or other medical problems.
- Muscle cramps, restless leg pain, itchy skin, and sores due to circulatory problems or vitamin D deficiency.
- Fibromyalgia.
- Complex Regional Pain Syndrome (CRPS), which develops after an illness or injury and often affects the leg, arm, foot, or hand.
- Injuries, especially from falls.

- *As we age, pain becomes a more common problem* due to the high prevalence of chronic and progressive pain-producing conditions associated with aging. It is estimated that up to 50% of older persons living in the community have pain that interferes with normal function, and 59–80% of nursing-home residents experience persistent pain [2, 3]. Alarmingly, being older than 70 is the leading risk factor for inadequate pain management [4].
- *Pain perceptions may change.* Alterations to somatic receptors that respond to touch, pressure, heat, cold, and pain may make patients less sensitive to pain

with advancing age. They may be less likely to report pain, have a higher threshold for pain, or feel less pain [5].

- *Use of certain medications in older patients becomes problematic* because of physiological changes [6]. Age-related changes, including reduced renal excretion and hepatic metabolism, can result in increased heightened drug sensitivity and adverse reactions to certain pain medications. Polypharmacy is also a contributing factor, as is the reluctance on the part of many providers to prescribe opioid pain medications.
- *Communication problems complicate diagnoses and treatment plans.* Older persons who have problems communicating – for example, from dementia or other mental impairments – are at greater risk of undertreatment of pain [7, 8].

For many people, navigating the health system and filling out complicated claim forms can be a dizzying misadventure. In order to overcome these problems, any forms or educational materials that are given to older adults should meet minimum health literacy requirements. Health literacy is "the degree to which individuals have the capacity to obtain, process, and understand basic health information and services needed to make appropriate health decisions," as defined by the National Library of Medicine and used in Healthy People 2010. For example, health literacy experts advise that health education materials use:

- Language that is at the 6–8th grade reading level
- Ten point or larger type size
- Adequate space between letters, lines, and paragraphs
- Colors that provide good contrast for easy reading
- Illustrations to convey complicated medical information

NIH-supported research is underway to develop and test technology programs that can be adapted for the elder chronic-care patient population in the home setting [9]. Online resources are evolving to provide resources that are "elder-friendly." One good example is the NIH Senior Health web site, http://nihseniorhealth.gov. This site is equipped with features to accommodate limited literacy levels, cognitive and physical impairments, and different modes of learning (e.g., textual, visual, auditory). Attempts to create accessible, easy-to-understand health information should be replicated in nonelectronic mediums. Just as care is taken to use pain assessment tools that are easy to follow, clinicians should also make sure that the information patients receive can be easily understood and used to make informed health decisions.

- *Access to quality pain care is often difficult* for patients because of the limited number of pain specialists and the fragmented U.S. health-care system, which often places the burden of care on individuals or families. Those 65 years of age and older often present with multiple medical and nutritional problems, take multiple medications, and have many potential sources of pain. This necessitates more coordinated care and planning.
- *Effective and supportive networks are critical as advanced age approaches, particularly for those living with pain and other chronic conditions.* This support network will depend somewhat on whether the patient is living independently at home but dependent on family, or residing in a retirement or planned community- assisted

living or long-term care. Each of these settings has unique challenges that must be considered. Geographic location can also influence the burden of care. Someone living in a rural community with few medical resources may feel isolated. The more isolated the elder, the more challenging their pain care becomes.

It should be noted that there is growing appeal to the "aging in place" concept, that is, allowing elders to live at home or in their communities rather than opting for institutional-based care. As more patients remain in their home environment, it is important that their health needs are addressed, including timely identification of pain problems and corresponding access to appropriate pain care.

- *Elders are vulnerable to potential discrimination.* Discrimination, which may be based on differences due to age, ability, gender, race, ethnicity, religion, sexual orientation, or any other characteristic by which people differ, can interfere with access to appropriate pain care and quality disease management and carry negative ramifications for health. Professional societies, including the American Nurses Association (ANA), are committed to working toward eradicating discrimination and racism with the medical profession and in education and training programs [10].

Pain is especially challenging among older adults due to persisting misperceptions, physiological changes that impact pain perception and usefulness of some pharmacological therapies, access to integrated pain management, and other issues. We know pain can be treated, and unmanaged pain needlessly compromises patients' quality of life. It is critical for clinicians to give older patients and their caregivers a road map with strategies to help negotiate their pain care and feel more in control of their health and well-being.

Advocating for Care

More and more we are realizing are realizing that when patients actively participate in their care, they fare better than those who take a passive, obedient role. In doing so, patients feel more in charge of their pain care, and tend to make treatment decisions with their health team that align with their lifestyle and preferences. They may be more adherent to recommended treatment strategies as well. Health-care professionals should take steps to promote patient education and self-advocacy to help improve treatment outcomes.

Patient education should be a priority. Clinicians should take the time to help older adults and their caregivers become educated consumers of pain management options. This includes understanding the specific pain condition, the goals of therapy, methods for pain assessment, appropriate use of pain medications, and self-help techniques. Patients use a variety of sources for health information. Age is one of the most important factors affecting health status, information-seeking, and media and Internet use, according to the National Institutes of Health [11]. A recent Pew Internet & Family Life Project survey found that eight in ten internet users look for health information online and that number continues to grow, even among seniors. Of these, over half (60%) report that their online searches influenced treatment decisions, and nearly 40% said that it influences their decision to see a doctor or not.

There are millions of health-related web sites that cater to the growing demand for medical information. But not all web sites are created equal. Some may contain false or misleading information. That is why it is important to learn about the site and determine whether the information is accurate and trustworthy. See APF's web site for *Top Ten Tips for Finding Quality Health Information Online*, a helpful resource for patients and families. If patients do not have access to the Internet at home, they may be able to find a computer with online access at their local library, public university, or senior center. Some of these venues now hold tutorials about how to start your search. Children, grandchildren, neighbors, and friends can also help research health information for them.

Of course, as even more people turn to online sources, many older people still rely on traditional information sources – talking to their doctor about health concerns, reading books, and conferring with friends and family members.

Finding personal support is essential for anyone living with pain, but especially for those entering advanced ages. Pairing older patients with pain champions and directing them to accessible and appropriate support networks can help ensure that they receive the pain care they deserve. This is critical to help them live the remainder of their lives with dignity and comfort.

Consider Helping Older Patients

- *Recruit a trusted family member or friend.* Encourage patients to find a "pain pal" to accompany them to appointments. This person can serve as a backup memory bank, write down answers to questions and concerns, and review instructions given during each visit. A "pain pal" can monitor and take note of what occurs after the visit and serve as a personal pain coach in their home environment. Remind patients to authorize that this person can receive confidential information, according to HIPPA rulings – they may be listed as one of the emergency contacts and should be encouraged to report any problems that occur in between office visits.
- *Assemble an interdisciplinary pain team.* Individuals with pain frequently report that this task requires "due diligence" and some element of luck to find the right providers. They see multiple providers before finding someone with the skills and willingness to treat their pain. Older adults typically do not have the time or extra energy to expend. As clinicians, we should help provide these patients with the resources and recommendations for building and sustaining an interdisciplinary pain team that can carefully coordinate care and necessary follow-up. Providing continuity of care will require practice settings and local communities to collaborate with one another.

- *Advocate for their care.* Part of our professional role is to serve as health advocates to our community and our patients. Recruiting the aid of an ombudsman, social worker, or other counselors at a local hospital, senior center, or long-term care facility for additional help can be a useful tactic when complex matters arise.

Advocacy is the cornerstone to excellence in patient care. Health-care professionals have not only an obligation, but also the privilege to serve as an advocate for their patients, many of whom, because of their age, medical condition, or mental health, may be unable to advocate for themselves. In addition, health-care providers are uniquely poised to serve as experts to inform policy and the news agenda.
The core domains of advocacy are the ability to work on behalf of or with:

- An individual
- An institution or community
- The public arena through educational awareness, social and political activities [12]

- *Link up with local and online patient support programs.* These support services can be found through hospitals, clinics, or national patient organizations such as the American Pain Foundation. Research and become familiar with online and local peer support programs that are suited for older patients and their caregivers. Keep an updated list handy to share with patients that includes:

- In-person support groups. Led and coordinated by individuals who live with pain or health-care professionals, typically social workers, nurses, or psychologists. These face-to-face meetings give patients and caregivers a regular place to come together and share challenges, fears, and successes in managing chronic pain and regaining quality of life. For more information, see the American Chronic Pain Association, http://www.theacpa.org/about/groups. asp Pain Connections, http://www.painconnection.org.
- Online Peer Support. Moderated by trained volunteers and health-care professionals. *PainAid*, APF's free online community featuring interactive discussion boards and chat rooms that are available 24/7 at http://painaid. painfoundation.org/. Here, peers actively provide support, information, and self-advocacy ideas. Health-care professional volunteers often assist with responses to specific medical questions, provide general information, and identify where visitors can get more detailed information. PainAid is a source of camaraderie and connectivity for those who prefer electronic communication options or need to reach out at any time.

- *Encourage those with pain to stand proud.* Engage and teach older patients how to balance speaking up about their pain experience, while respecting their preference for keeping their health issues a private matter. This might prove to be challenging with some patients who prefer not to change their ways, but it is important to give them the encouragement to speak up about the pain they experience and how it affects their daily lives.

Rights to Care, Pain Management, and Health Coverage Laws

The ethical tenet of autonomy supports pain management as a basic human right. Patients [of all ages] have a right to receive optimal pain relief and be involved in their pain management treatment plan. The patient has a right to be informed of pain management treatments, benefits and risks of procedures, alternative pain management modalities, and expected outcomes [13]. Notable experts have stated that "inadequate pain treatment is an entrenched problem around the world, related to cultural, societal, religious, and political factors…[which is tantamont to] the acceptance of torture" [14]. It is imperative that clinicians honor their professional duty by ensuring that our vulnerable patients, like elders with pain, are aware of their rights to pain relief and quality of care. We must act on their behalf accordingly.

One aspect of providing quality care is becoming familiar with the laws that help protect you and your patients. These laws are designed to protect patients' basic rights or extend health coverage due to change or loss of coverage or employment. Patient Bill of Rights (see example below), HIPPA, COBRA, ERISA, and the Women's Health and Cancer Rights Act are just a few.

Pain Care Bill of Rights

As a person with pain, you have the right to:
- Have your report of pain taken seriously and to be treated with dignity and respect by doctors, nurses, pharmacists, social workers, and other health-care professionals.
- Have your pain thoroughly assessed and promptly treated.
- Participate actively in decisions about how to manage your pain.
- Be informed and know your options: talk with your health-care provider about your pain – possible cause(s), treatment options, and the benefits, risks, and costs of each choice.
- Have your pain reassessed regularly and your treatment adjusted if your pain has not been eased.
- Be referred to a pain specialist if your pain persists.
- Get clear and prompt answers to your questions, take time to make decisions, and refuse a particular type of treatment if you choose.

  Although not always required by law, these are the rights
  you should expect for your pain care.
  Courtesy American Pain Foundation

Transition of Care

Intentional or unintentional abandonment of patients with pain is a growing concern for many who practice pain management. This can be devastating and life-threatening for our elder population, no matter the reason. Developing a relationship with a new health-care provider is difficult for most, and highly stressful for our elders, especially if they have had a long-term relationship with the former health-care provider. The disruption of continuity of care can set the stage for a rapid deterioration of their baseline health status and can be compounded if access to required medications that modify pain are withdrawn or severely limited. Medically unsupervised withdrawal from opiates, benzodiazepines, some antidepressants, and steroids can cause premature death, especially in our frail elder population.

By law and by ethics, health-care professionals cannot abandon their patients. We are obligated to arrange for the transition of care for our established patients. Yet abandonment happens. One example is when a practice is closed due to relocation or retirement: another provider or group may either purchase that business practice or make an agreement to accept those patients into their practice. Patient records are then transferred to that new practice. This implies that the medical relationship is transferred as well. The patient should be provided official notice of those arrangements and given the option to continue care with that new practice or directed to other providers to arrange for transfer of care.

If the new provider is unable or unwilling to manage their pain, a referral to a pain specialist or another primary-care provider should be arranged. Referrals to pain specialists most frequently require a physician request and transfer of medical information. Referral lists may be prepared and provided by the individual practice, or the patient could be instructed to obtain one through the area hospitals or the medical licensing board in that state. These lists are limited at best. They often do not list if the provider has expertise or interest in pain management, whether he is in primary care or a specialist – much less someone with expertise in geriatric pain management. Finding a practitioner who accepts new patients, accepts a variety of insurance plans, and has a waiting list of under 30 days is a tall order for most.

Continued care, until a referral has been completed and the patient has been accepted into a new practice, remains an obligation of the medical provider who may not be interested in providing pain care during that gap in transfer. While the transfer of care is delayed due to long wait times for new appointments etc., the stigma of being a patient with pain is reinforced – unfair labeling as an unwanted patient. This is rarely replicated in other chronic diseases, such as diabetes or cardiac disease. The commonality seems to fall with those who live with mental illness or addictive disease. This is particularly an unfair burden to our elder population.

Far worse is when the appropriate transfer of care does not occur. This is equivalent to medical abandonment. Behaviors have been reported that patients with pain [no matter the age, no matter the cause] have been sent a certified letter that they no longer have care within 30 days, some have final prescription(s) issued, others do not; some have not successfully secured access to a new provider. Further action could be warranted as a necessary next step, such as filing reports to State Boards of Medicine, hospital ethics committees, state and federal legislators, and policy makers, as well as the local news media.

Transition of care, no matter the reason, should be a well-planned process, particularly for our elder population. Coordination may be required, with the support of nursing, social work, insurance provider, and respective health-care providers involved in the transition.

Overcoming Myths Stereotypes and Misunderstandings

In addition, common misconceptions about pain may stand in the way of appropriate pain management.

Common Misperceptions about Pain

Pain is complex and frequently misunderstood by the public. The issue of pain is riddled with myths and misperceptions, which makes the task of informing and educating people about pain and its management that much more challenging.

Some myths about pain from APF's the American Pain Foundation Reporter's Guide:

Pain is "all in your head." Although this is partially true because we need our brains for the perception of pain, that does not mean pain is imaginary when the source of pain is not well understood. Pain is all too real to the person who lives with it day in, day out.

Pain is just something one has to live with – an inevitable part of a disease or condition. The fact is that most pain can be relieved with proper pain management.

Pain is a natural part of growing older. While pain is more common as we age because conditions that cause pain (e.g., arthritis, degenerative joint diseases, cancer, shingles, osteoporosis) are more frequent in older adults, it should not be something people have to struggle with.

The best judge of pain is the physician or nurse. Studies have shown that there is little correlation between what a physician or nurse might "guess" about someone's actual pain. The person with pain is the authority on the existence and severity of his/her pain. The self-report is the most reliable indicator.

Seeking medical care for pain is a sign of weakness. Pain carries a stigma, and many people hesitate talking about their pain and how it affects their daily life; they also do not want to be considered a "bad" patient.

Use of strong pain medication leads to addiction. Many people living with pain and even some health-care providers falsely believe opioids (strong pain medicines) are universally addictive. Studies have shown that the risk of addiction is small when these medicines are properly prescribed and taken as directed. As with any medication, there are risks, but these risks can be managed.

Source: American Pain Foundation, A Reporter's Guide: Covering Pain and Its Management at www.painfoundation.org under the Newsroom tab.

Tips for Self-care

It is important that older patients and their loved ones understand that they can advocate for quality pain management. The first step is to ensure that patients understand that pain is not an inevitable part of growing older and that there are a variety of pharmacologic and nonpharmacologic options for managing pain and improving function.

There are many self-care strategies that people living with pain can use to help improve their health outcomes. By playing an active role in managing pain, patients and their loved ones will feel enabled to influence their treatment and improve their health and well-being. Some of these steps have been mentioned earlier but deserve repeating.

1. *Assemble a competent, interdisciplinary health-care team.* Because the older patient population is more likely to suffer with multiple chronic conditions as well as adverse reactions to pain relievers and other medications, it is critical to provide a holistic, team approach to care. Treatment plans must be carefully coordinated, and all members of the health team should stay informed about the patient's condition, applied therapies, and associated improvements or worsening of function and quality of life.
2. *Keep a pain journal.* Pain is a subjective experience and unique to each individual. Patients' self-reports of pain provide health professionals with the most insight into the nature and intensity of pain. Because pain can interfere with sleep, mood, and overall quality of life, it is important that patients track their pain (when it occurs, for how long, the level and type of pain, possible triggers, etc.), its impact on daily routines and mobility, and their response to various treatments over time, including any troublesome side effects and noticeable improvements in physical function and emotional wellness.

   Patients can easily record this information using the American Pain Foundation's Targeting Chronic Pain Notebook available at http://www.painfoundation.org/Publications/TargetNotebook.pdf. This resource can also help facilitate ongoing communication with their health-care providers.
3. *Get enough sleep.* Just as sleep promotes healing, not getting enough can be physically and emotionally draining, often worsening pain and depression. As we get older, the body makes fewer chemicals and hormones that help us sleep well and sleep disorders such as restless leg syndrome, insomnia, and periodic limb movement can spell trouble when it comes to restorative sleep. Make sure to encourage patients to adopt better nighttime habits (also known as sleep hygiene):

   (a) Try to get 7–8 h of sleep each night.
   (b) Go to bed and wake up at the same time everyday.
   (c) Create a calming ritual by taking a warm bath/shower, meditating, reading or listening to calming music.
   (d) Use comfortable bedding and sleepwear.
   (e) Keep the bedroom cool, dark, and quiet.

(f) Go to bed at the same time every night.
(g) Use the bedroom for sleep and intimacy only; unplug the TV.
(h) Limit caffeine and alcohol; avoid food at least 4 h before retiring.
(i) Forgo long daytime naps.

Some people may need a sleep aid to help get restorative sleep.

4. *Stay mentally and physically active.* People living with pain will often avoid certain movements or activities, fearing they will cause a painful response. They may also refrain from socializing, pursuing hobbies, even leaving the house because of the sheer anxiety or anticipation of being overcome with a pain flare. Still, patients should try to stay as engaged as possible to stay connected and use their mind – whether it is doing crosswords or picking up a new hobby to help sharpen their minds.

5. *Manage stress.* When the body endures prolonged periods of stress, it is flooded with stress chemicals that can trigger painful flare-ups. While stress, depression, and anxiety do not cause chronic pain, they do commonly coexist with pain. Pain, in turn, can interfere with concentration, mood, and ability to cope with stress. It becomes a vicious cycle.

Many patients benefit from incorporating *relaxation techniques* that help to relieve muscle tension, cope with stress, and reduce pain sensations. It is also important to advise patients to steer clear of harmful habits (e.g., consuming too much caffeine, smoking, overindulging in food), which can exacerbate pain. Instead, engaging in gentle exercise or relaxing pastimes and eating a balanced diet can help.

6. *Strengthen relationships.* Pain can lead to feelings of isolation and loneliness. Many patients withdraw from social activities, which can have an adverse affect on them and their loved ones. Open communication and achieving a common understanding of the impact of pain can complement medical therapy.

7. *Maintain a healthy sense of humor.* It is not always easy for people to stay upbeat when they are in pain. But, an optimistic outlook can not only improve mood but may also strengthen the immune system. There is increasing emphasis on "humor therapy" and its role in healing. Studies suggest a good laugh can alleviate stress and depression and promote relaxation by lowering blood pressure and improving breathing and muscle function. Best of all, laughter is a low-cost, effective form of mood management that is accessible to everyone. So, patients should be encouraged to spend time with their grandchildren, share a joke with a neighbor, rent their favorite comedy, and generally look for the humor and the "upside" of everyday life.

8. *Pay attention to good nutrition.* Many people who have lived with pain feel that their energy levels have been depleted. Eating well is essential to good health and can be a good stress reducer as well. Patients should:

(a) Avoid caffeine, alcohol, and sugar – they can irritate muscles and increase stress. If you drink a lot of coffee, tea, or soda, talk with your doctor about how to lower your intake slowly so that you do not have symptoms of caffeine withdrawal (e.g., headaches or nausea).

(b) Eat a well-balanced diet that includes lots of fresh fruits and vegetables, lean meats, and whole grains.

(c) Stay hydrated by drinking lots of fluids.

(d) Beware of "miracle diets" that claim to treat fibromyalgia or other pain conditions after fibro. Some supplements and foods may cause serious side effects when mixed with certain medications.

9. *Seek support*. Patients should not feel as though they have to cope with pain alone. It is important that they talk openly with trusted friends and family members about how they are feeling, and not be afraid to ask for help when it is needed.

   Online or local support groups can help patients connect with others who are facing similar challenges. These groups provide a forum for people living with pain. PainAid, APF's online support community, is available around the clock, http://painaid.painfoundation.org/. Some patients may benefit from counseling or other psychosocial support.

10. *Call on others for help*. Having a trusted friend or family member, who can help their loved one navigate the health-care system, understand his or her pain condition, tell them how best to adhere to treatment protocols, and serve as their personal cheerleader in times of doubt, is important.

APF offers a wealth of support services, booklets, newsletters, expert Q&As, and other print- and Web-based materials designed to meet the unique needs of people living with pain, their caregivers, and health providers.

Resources for Older People with Pain

The following, while not an exhaustive list, provides useful resources for helping patients to navigate the health-care system, access quality care advocacy resources with information about filing complaints and finding legal resources, tools for caregivers and general health and aging topics, research, and publications.

Navigating the Health Care System

Tap a social worker. In the last decade, the national social workers' associations have informed their membership about pain, its management, and the role of social workers. They have been actively engaged in the pain and palliative care movement. The nature of their work demonstrates their commitment to help others find their way from access to care to living their final days with dignity. There are two prominent organizations ready to serve:

- National Association of Social Work has a professional locator at: http://www.helpstartshere.org/common/Search/Default.asp
- Association of Oncology Social Work has a patient and family resource link: http://www.aosw.org/html/patfam-resources.php

American Pain Foundation

http://www.painfoundation.org

APF is working to improve the quality of life of people with pain by raising public awareness, providing practical information, promoting research, and advocating removal of barriers and increased access to effective pain management. APF has a wide range of online and print materials for people living with pain and their loved ones. A few helpful resources include:

Access matters: Understanding your health coverage booklet provides general information about various types of health insurance and programs, things to consider when comparing health plans, how to protect and get the most from health coverage, and resources to advocate for oneself.

Pain resource locator is an online searchable database that links visitors to disease-specific organizations that can provide the information, support, and resources needed to manage pain. Categories include prescription drug assistance, insurance and benefits, caregiver resources among many others. See http://www. painfoundation.org/ResourceLocator.asp.

Pain resource guide: Getting the help you need. Whether someone has started experiencing pain or has lived with it for years, they are bound to have lots of questions. This 32-page booklet provides an overview of pain, its assessment, and treatment. It also gives readers tips for taking an active role on the road to pain relief, including how to find a pain specialist and online or local support services, questions to ask health-care providers, and strategies to cope with pain.

Treatment options: A guide for people living with pain. Making sound medical decisions rests heavily on knowing what treatment options are available. This booklet gives readers an overview of different options for pain management. Written and reviewed by leading pain specialists, this guide provides credible, comprehensive information about medications, psychosocial interventions, complementary approaches, rehabilitation therapies, surgical interventions, and more.

Quality Care Advocacy Resources

Medicare Quality Improvement Organizations (QIOs, formally known as Peer Review Organizations or PROs). By law (under Sections 1152–1154 of the Social Security Act), the mission of the QIO Program is to improve the effectiveness, efficiency, economy, and quality of services delivered to Medicare beneficiaries. Based on this statutory charge, and the Center for Medicare and Medicaid Services (CMS) experience, CMS identifies the core functions of the QIO Program as:

- Improving quality of care for beneficiaries.
- Protecting the integrity of the Medicare Trust Fund by ensuring that Medicare pays only for services and goods that are reasonable and necessary and that are provided in the most appropriate setting.

- Protecting beneficiaries by expeditiously addressing individual complaints, such as beneficiary complaints; provider-based notice appeals; violations of the Emergency Medical Treatment and Labor Act (EMTALA); and other related responsibilities as articulated in QIO-related law [15].

QIO organizations are required to conduct reviews of written complaints filed by Medicare beneficiaries about the quality of medical services that were received. Letters should be addressed to the specific QIO assigned to the geographic area where the problem occurred. The QIO Directory (Quality Net) can be found online at: http:// www.qualitynet.org/dcs/ContentServer?pagename=Medqic/MQGeneralPage/ GeneralPageTemplate&name=QIO%20Listings

Citizen Advocacy Center

http://www.cacenter.org
   The Citizen Advocacy Center (CAC) has an ongoing initiative to improve the way pain is treated and managed in the U.S. CAC is a not-for-profit training and advocacy organization with a special mission to train and support public members who serve on state health licensing boards (e.g., boards of medicine, nursing, pharmacy, physical therapy) to make them more effective in protecting and promoting the public interest. This is accomplished through networking preparing issue papers, convening an annual educational forum, developing special training and policy development forums on selected issues, among other coordinated activities. CAC assists the public with filing complaints to regulatory agencies, such as Boards of Medicine, Pharmacy, Nursing, etc., when poor pain management has been an issue or breach of professional duty, such as abandonment, has been identified.

National Long-Term Care Ombudsmen Resource Center

http://www.ltcombudsman.org/static_pages/ombudsmen.cfm
   Ombudsmen advocate for residents' rights and quality care, educate consumers and providers, resolve complaints, and provide information to the public to enhance quality of life.. Under the federal Older Americans Act, every state is required to have an Ombudsman Program that addresses complaints and advocates for improvements in the long-term-care system. Quality pain care is on their radar screen. They are trained to resolve problems and can assist you with complaints. However, the patient or designee must give the ombudsman permission to share his or her concerns, which are kept confidential.

Administration on Aging Resources: Eldercare Locator

http://www.eldercare.gov

AoA's mission is to help elderly individuals maintain their dignity and independence in their homes and communities through comprehensive, coordinated, and cost-effective systems of long-term care, and livable communities across the U.S.

Patient Advocate Association

http://www.patientadvocate.org

A national nonprofit organization that seeks to safeguard patients through effective mediation, assuring access to care, maintenance of employment, and preservation of their financial stability relative to their diagnosis of life-threatening or debilitating diseases.

Elder Law: Legal Resources

Elder Law Answers

http://www.elderlawanswers.com

Elder Law Answers supports seniors, their families, and their attorneys in achieving their goals by providing quality information on the Internet about crucial legal issues facing seniors and an online practice tool for elder law attorneys. An attorney locator resource is provided; attorneys listed in the network affirm that they have demonstrated a commitment to the field of elder law.

Caregiver Resources

Eldercare at Home

Chapter 11 – Pain, by the American Geriatric Society is a free comprehensive online guide for family caregivers; this chapter offers a problem-solving approach to managing pain at home and working cooperatively with health-care providers. http//:www.healthinaging.org/public_education/eldercare/11.xml

Assessing pain in older adults with dementia is a brochure for family members and other caregivers that provides advice from the experts. http//:www.healthinaging.org/public_education/pain/pain_dementia_v4.pdf.

General Health and Aging

American Geriatrics Society

http//:www.americangeriatrics.org
  AGS is devoted to improving the health, independence, and quality of life of all older people. The Society provides leadership to health-care professionals, policy makers, and the public by implementing and advocating for programs in patient care, research, professional and public education, and public policy.
Aging in the know: Your gateway to health and aging resources on the Web. Aging in the Know offers up-to-date information for consumers on health and aging. http//:www.healthinaging.org/agingintheknow/

Centers for Disease Control and Prevention: Healthy Aging for Older Adults

http//:www.cdc.gov/aging
  The web site features publications on the state of health and aging in America; preventing disease and increasing quality of life among older adults; information on caregiving; tools for patients and caregivers; list of CDC-funded research programs; and links to related organizations

National Institute on Aging

http//:www.nia.nih.gov/healthinformation/
  The web site provides information and tips on healthy aging, caregiving, medications, dietary supplements, and diseases; clinical trials; and an online, searchable database with more than 300 national organizations that provide help to older people.

Alzheimer's Association

http//:www.alz.org
  The Alzheimer's Association is the leading voluntary health organization in Alzheimer care, support, and research. The organization is working to eliminate Alzheimer's disease through the advancement of research; to provide and enhance care and support for all who are affected; and to reduce the risk of dementia through the promotion of brain health.

Women's Institute for a Secure Retirement (WISER)

http://www.wiserwomen.org/portal/index.php?option=com_content&task=view&id=348&Itemid=52
Full listing of health and aging resources for minorities and diverse populations.

References

1. Weiner DK, Rudy TE. Attitudinal barriers to effective treatment of persistent pain in nursing home residents. J Am Geriatr Soc. 2002;50(12):2035–40.
2. Ferrell BA. Pain evaluation and management in the nursing home. Ann Intern Med. 1995;123:681–7.
3. Helme RD, Gibson SJ. Pain in older people. In: Crombie IK, editor. Epidemiology of pain. Seattle: IASP Press; 1999. p. 103–12.
4. Cleeland, CS, Gonin R, Hatfield AK, Edmonson JH, Blum RH, Stewart JA, et al. Pain and its treatment in outpatients with metastatic cancer. N Engl J Med. 1994;330(9):592–6.
5. Ferrini AF, Ferrini RL. Health in the later years. 3rd ed. Boston, MA: McGraw Hill; 2000.
6. Parmalee PA, Smith B, Katz IR. Pain complaints and cognitive status among elderly institution residents. J Am Geriatr Soc. 1992;41:517–22.
7. Schmucker DL. Liver function and phase I drug metabolism in the elderly: a paradox. Drugs Aging. 2001;18:837–51.
8. Malloy DC, Hadjistavropoulos T. The problem of pain management among persons with dementia, personhood, and the ontology of relationships. Nurs Philos. 2004;5(2):147–59.
9. Kaufman DL, Patel VL, Hilliman C, Morin PC, Pevzner J, Weinstock RS, Goland R, et al. Usability in the real world: assessing medical information technologies in patients' homes. J Biomed Inform. 2003;36:45–60.
10. ANA. Position Statement: Discrimination and Racism in Health Care – March 1998. http://www.nursingworld.org/MainMenuCategories/HealthcareandPolicyIssues/ANAPosition Statements/EthicsandHumanRights.aspx. Accessed July 2009.
11. U.S. Department of Health and Human Services, Office of Disease Prevention and Health Promotion. "Mapping Diversity to Understand Users' Requirements for e-Health Tools" in "Expanding the Reach and Impact of Consumer e-Health Tools" Chapter 2. June 2006. Available at http://www.health.gov/communication/ehealth/ehealthTools/chapter2_part2.htm.
12. Lewis J, Arnold MS, House R, Toporek R. Advocacy competencies [Electronic version]. 2003. Retrieved October 3, 2006. http://www.counseling.org/Publications. Accessed July 2009.
13. Ferrell B. Ethical perspectives on pain and suffering. Pain Manag Nurs. 2005;6(3):83–90.
14. Brennan F, Carr DB, Cousins M. Pain management: a fundamental human right. Anesth Analg. 2007;105:205–21.
15. Center for Medicare and Medicaid Services (CMS). Overview of Medicare Quality Improvement. http://www.cms.hhs.gov/QualityImprovementOrgs/. Accessed July 2009.

Chapter 14
Suggestions for Change: Education, Policy, and Communication

F. Michael Gloth, III

> *Greatness is not in where we stand, but in what direction we are moving. We must sail sometimes with the wind, and sometimes against it – but sail we must, and not drift, nor lie at anchor.*

> Oliver Wendell Holmes

Everyone should have access to affordable, convenient, and effective assessment and pain management. The concepts for improving pain management in our society encompass three broad areas, education, policy, and communication. This is not to ignore reimbursement. However, because of the Federal and State involvement with Medicare and Medicaid, real changes in compensation for pain care reside in policy changes, and most of these are fundamentally with the Centers for Medicare and Medicaid Services (CMS), a part of the Department of Health and Human Services. Since most insurance carriers model off of reimbursement rates and strategies from CMS, that seems to be the most logical place to start the wheels of change into motion.

The other area that clearly needs additional effort is research. For practical reasons, that has been included in both education and policy discussions. Research on pain is done predominantly through grants in academic settings or by industry. Both are strongly affected by initiatives outlined in the sections of this chapter on education and policy.

It should be recognized that a worrisome change has occurred in recent years that has jeopardized education and research. There has been a steady deterioration in the relationship between academic medicine and industry. Despite huge efforts to accommodate concerns about bias and undue influence from industry, the academic medical community, in particular, has been on a crusade to vilify industry with almost a laser-like focus on the pharmaceutical industry. As a consequence, many educational programs and industry-sponsored research have been unintended casualties.

F.M. Gloth, III (✉)
Division of Geriatric Medicine and Gerontology, Johns Hopkins University School of Medicine, Baltimore, MD, USA
e-mail: fgloth1@jhmi.edu

F.M. Gloth, III (ed.), *Handbook of Pain Relief in Older Adults: An Evidence-Based Approach*, Aging Medicine, DOI 10.1007/978-1-60761-618-4_14,
© Springer Science+Business Media, LLC 2011

The pharmacy industry has responded to every accusation, whether justified or not. As a consequence, there is full disclosure of emoluments to health care professionals who consult with, speak for, or advise pharmaceutical companies. Continuing Medication Education programs have full disclosures of potential conflicts of interest, even remote ones. Independent panels have been established for the assignment of grants and speaker's bureaus. Unprecedented efforts have gone forward to ensure that speakers do not breach Food and Drug restrictions on promotional programs. Many academic programs have gone so far as to restrict employees from participating in such roles, even outside of their employment time! Bureaucracy for speakers has increased and CME paperwork has become onerous enough to have many organizations abandon such programs completely. Despite all of these restrictions, pharmaceutical sales have exceeded prior records, the industry continues to provide more research than all National Institute on Health (NIH) institutes combined.

Arguably, academics have suffered as many faculty members are no longer well versed with respect to upcoming developments in the pharmaceutical field. It appears that ignorance may not be the solution after all, as we see educational and research projects from community educational organizations suffering from, what has been perceived by some, as an adversarial relationship between health care professionals and the pharmaceutical industry. The pendulum may have swung so far that the bias is predominantly on the side of the academic professionals and professional journal editorial boards who allow selected advertising, but cast a jaundiced eye toward colleagues who interact with the pharmaceutical industry. In a recent article about the pharmaceutical industry's interaction with physician, some physicians were listed as being authors without substantially contributing or writing articles or for contracting for articles with pharmaceutical companies. The implication was that such health care professionals were simply allowing their names to be used, without contributing or perhaps even agreeing with the content. Amazingly, the authors of the article did not even have a discussion with the authors or even make an effort to ascertain whether such relationships truly existed, and this was published in one of the most widely circulated journals in the world [1]! It appears that evidence-based information is not reliably available, regardless of the source. Conflicts and biases exist at all levels and the ancient warning, "Caveat emptor," applies in every setting. For this reason and many others, progress on education and research remains a priority.

This chapter addresses suggestions that have feasible solutions. It does not deal with concepts that are not currently practical or politically viable.

Education

Every health care professional school, especially medical, nursing, and pharmacy school, in the USA needs to add further, more standardized instruction on pain management and end-of-life (or hospice) care into the curriculum [2]. Certainly, we can do better than the dismal performance of medical schools with such programs at present [3]. Since every medical practitioner, with only a few exceptions like pathologists, will confront pain patients on a regular basis, this would only make sense, even at the sacrifice of some other areas of instruction. So too, the topic of pain management should be formally covered in most medical residency training programs.

It should be recognized that in order to accomplish this goal, there would need to be adequate instructors available to provide this recommended instruction. Currently, there are not. This means that Continuing Medical Education (CME) courses will be necessary for many of the medical faculty who would be involved in this process.

Efforts to provide CME training to a large number of health care professionals in practice have been difficult to maintain. The Maryland End-of Life Training (MET) Program through the Hospice Network of Maryland was a program that worked with physician leaders, who had received additional training modeled on the American Medical Association's Education for Physicians on End-of-life Care (EPEC) Project. These physicians would then go throughout the State, speaking in hospital grand rounds settings. Funding issues led to the demise of this program.

Recognizing the need to identify folks with expertise the concept of Board Certification has expanded to hospice and other areas related to pain management. Some organizations focusing on pain offer additional credentialing in pain management. Unfortunately, the certification process has lost some of its histori- cally hallowed stature. In recent years, there has been a movement to require recer- tification of individuals. While this has increased the cost, time, and resources that individuals must expend to maintain certification, there have been some disturbing trends associated with the practice. Most people who participate in the process oversight are themselves conflicted. Many belong to organizations that profit by conducting board preparations courses. Some individuals receive important com- pensation for their oversight efforts, either directly or indirectly. Amazingly, there are no data that indicate that anyone who received initial certification in any field and continues to work in the field with CMEs being taken in the area, performs any better or provides any better care if they get recertified than their colleagues who do not. Nonetheless, regulatory agencies, insurance companies, and various other organizations (e.g., hospitals) gauge acceptance based on such certification and recertification. The only thing that is assured by such recertification is that the recertified physician has spent hundreds, if not thousands, of dollars on test costs, review courses, and time away from the office for taking and preparing for the test itself. In a time of terrible shortages in physician supply, it is almost unconscionable to place such demands on practitioners without evidence of merit [4].

Despite the concern about the status of "Board Certification," it is a reality. To emphasize the importance of education on pain relief among professionals, testing to obtain licensure or board certification should include questions on pain manage- ment scenarios. This will assure that pain relief instruction has an appropriate place at the table of medical learning.

Educational efforts will need to be directed to the public as well. This effort will need to be augmented by a plan for communicating to the public about the availability of such information and developing venues to promote and disseminate such information. Educational efforts should involve advertising, public symposia, articles, talk shows, the internet, and promotional efforts by government and private community-based health care entities. The local health care community along with the spiritual community also must support such efforts. Additionally, the business community needs to be supportive and facilitate the educational efforts, especially in light of the economic losses that are incurred due to pain. Such costs are not only from direct loss of an employee in pain, but also indirectly by an employee's relative in pain costing the healthy employee time away from work to help that relative.

Beyond health care professionals and the general public, an educational effort needs to target two other groups, i.e., legislators and policy makers, along with pain patients themselves. The important goal here is to provide a mechanism for such groups to be able to identify reliable information as opposed to the specious pieces, which will always be competing for attention. It is important to be proactive in getting such information to the appropriate people.

Funding for such educational efforts should come from private donors, better reimbursement for pain management, and government and industry grants. To do so the relationship between industry and the public and academic sectors needs to be more collegial.

Policy

Duplicate and triplicate prescriptions should be eliminated. Such practices have not been shown to have any substantial impact on illicit drug use, but do adversely affect prescribing and, thus, pain control [5]. An increase in opioid consumption does not correlate with an increase in drug deaths, but can be associated with better pain control [5]. Federal regulations should protect prescribers of pain medication even should that medication increase the risk of death or hasten death.

Punitive regulations regarding mandates on education should be eliminated or avoided. Such programs have yet to prove effective, are costly, and promote ill will towards a most noble cause. Rather, incentives, e.g., reductions in malpractice insurance rates, reduced medical society dues, improved reimbursement for demonstrating pain management competency and training makes more sense, and would be better embraced by the medical community.

Electronic medical record (EMR) systems that provide pain treatment guidance and prescription capability should be encouraged. Funding for demonstration products and outcome-based research of such systems is needed and should be part of the Request for Proposals program at the National Institutes of Health as well as other government-funded research programs. Practices that use EMR systems with the ability to reduce drug–drug interactions, facilitate communication, provide instant data retrieval, facilitate acquisition of information reduce adverse events, etc. should also receive reductions in malpractice insurance rates, reduced medical society dues, improved reimbursement as incentive for transitioning a busy office practice to such systems, which are also likely to improve quality of care and quality improvement practices [6, 7].

The American Association of Medical Colleges (AAMC) should continue to place emphasis on pain education, and focus less on demographic quotas and more on motivation for medical school. Primary care with an interest in hospice, geriatrics, and pain management should be targets of such selection processes for medical schools. Allowing more medical school slots rather than less would also be useful. Few have been impressed with the AAMC's ability to predict physician need. The Accreditation Council for Graduate Medical Education (ACGME) also needs to place greater emphasis on pain management and hospice in residency training programs. Efforts have been fairly anemic from this organization to date, particularly with regards to monitoring faculty competence and oversight.

Not only must reimbursement for pain management be increased, payment must occur in a timely fashion. Enrollment in such programs and credentialing processes must be streamlined. Currently, in the Baltimore area experience at Victory Springs Senior Health Associates has indicated that credentialing at facilities can cost hundreds of dollars per physician and take months to attain. Every bureaucratic obstacle delays improvements in care and compromises quality. In this age of information technology, there is no reason that this process cannot be streamlined, and no good reason that a standardized process cannot be implemented and perhaps sanctioned by legislation to assure an integrated translation of information to all credentialing bodies.

Few health care providers are not familiar with quality assurance (QA) or quality improvement (QI). Such terms are used under the presumption that quality of care and, thus, quality of life will be demonstrably better. Such aspirations are to be applauded, but at times the process supersedes the ultimate goals. Organizations participate in an accreditation process, practitioners obtain certification, and regulatory agencies conduct site visits and surveys. Sometimes this occurs paradoxically to the detriment of patient or resident care. Every certification, every accreditation, and every surveyor generate exorbitant costs. One would presume that any such certifying or credentialing body would hold themselves to an objective standard to assure internal quality. Interestingly, that is rarely the case. The Joint Committee on Accreditation of Healthcare Organizations has not demonstrated correlation with their scoring to hospital outcomes. There are no studies indicating that recertification identifies better practitioners than initial certification in a medical specialty, e.g., internal medicine or geriatrics. Rating systems for nursing homes are based on the federally mandated Minimum Data Set (MDS), and CMS itself has noted that their nursing home comparisons based on such scoring "...do not present a complete picture of the quality of care provided by the nursing home. The inspection measures whether the nursing home meets the minimum standard for a particular set of requirements. If a nursing home has no deficiencies, it means that it met the minimum standards at the time of the inspection. However, this information cannot be used to identify nursing homes that provide outstanding care [8]." States have also used such systems with the same lack of correlation. One example of a State's disclaimer notes that the "...scoring system, developed in collaboration with the nursing home industry and nursing home resident advocates, includes some self-declared and unverified information [9]."

All such organizations and certifying bodies should be required to demonstrate some association between measures and clinical outcomes. Amazingly, the literature is replete with "evidence-based" evaluations of guidelines, protocols, and recommendations. The same people who insist upon such stringent criteria overlook these same principals when it comes to assessing quality and measures of overall clinical care. Is it because of some inherent bias? Is it that a credentialing body is tied to an organization that profits from this process either directly through funds to the organization for writing, developing, and administering the tests or indirectly through the courses that are offered at their home institutions for test preparation? There does seem to be a tremendous conflict of interest at the very least. How can JCAHO accreditation be required for hospital licensure, if there are not data to demonstrate improved care associated with accreditation? JCAHO might offer data that facilities that perform better on State surveys are more likely to be JCAHO certified. Perhaps more conscientious facilities are also more market conscious and provide a better product regardless of certification, but are also more likely to seek certification in the first place.

Why is it that State survey results for commonly recognized "excellent" nursing homes are often indistinguishable from commonly recognized "unsatisfactory" facilities? Could it be that the survey process is time consuming, costly, and takes effort and resources away from patient or resident care? Could it be that the surveyors are inadequately experienced and inadequately staffed? Is it possible that some facilities work towards fulfilling survey requirements with loss of some attention on practical needs of the patient? For some facilities, there is a QI process for the State or accreditation bodies and separate QI focus on issues directed toward improving patient/resident care. These facilities are probably the best overall, but that will not be measured very well.

Regardless of the reasons considered above, regulations and certification or credentialing processes that do not demonstrate improved clinical outcomes should be revoked or at least publicly rejected. If every physician stopped sitting for recertification, the process would be recognized for the lack of relevance that has been demonstrated. There also would not be the financial incentive to continue and, subsequently, there would be a decline in recertification boards.

This is not to suggest that QA programs should be abandoned or that we should abandon effort towards QI. Research to identify prospectively, in a real-world setting quality measures that correlate consistently with clinical outcomes in relevant populations should be funded and encouraged. Perhaps more useful would be to provide people with expertise and training to oversee programs and facilities. These medical leaders should also have the authority to initiate changes directed at improving care and improving safety. Reimbursement also needs to be commensurate with the responsibility and commitment required to provide adequate oversight. The funding can come from the savings associated with the elimination of the plethora of inadequate regulatory, accreditation, and certification programs currently burdening the health care system. This would also allow a greater focus on pain management and pain instruction with rewards for better clinical outcomes, including pain relief.

Certainly, piloting such conceptual projects would make immense sense and may finally lead to some evidence-based changes in how we oversee pain management in older people in a variety of health care settings. There must also be additional vigilance for health system requirements that create an environment which makes pain management more difficult. Usually, such mandates come from government or other regulatory bodies. Usually such constraints are not intended to be harmful, but rather are based on a well-intentioned solution to another problem. The Drug Enforcement Agency (DEA) is particularly susceptible to such conflicts with solutions resulting in unintended adverse effects on pain relief efforts. For example, in 2009, administrative leadership at the DEA decided that the agency would begin to crack down on pharmacy providers of analgesics to nursing homes. Because nursing homes did not fit into the same category as hospitals, the method of prescribing certain types of drugs in the nursing home setting requires a different process. In prior years, however, this was recognized as being impractical and the DEA allowed nursing homes to have drugs ordered through the doctors order sheet and by phone order through the nurses as would happen in the hospital. The logic being that the enforcement of statute to require prescribers to write a prescription for every higher level pain drug (called Schedule II and later Schedule III–V were included) order would create an environment where nursing home residents would be unable to get needed pain relief in a timely fashion in that setting due to the increased complexities, paperwork, and time involved in such prescribing protocols. In 2009, the decision to enforce that law was made and, predictably, prescribers found themselves in just the predicament that was expected. At the time of this writing a patient who needs a new prescription for one of the stronger pain medications must have the physician call the pharmacy and order an initial prescription for the nurses to provide a medication from the supply in the nursing home. Another prescription is needed for an emergency supply that can be provided for only 3 days by phone. A third prescription for a longer interval must then be written and the originals for all sent to the pharmacy. All of this must then be relayed to the nursing staff to begin the process. Because the prescriber is often not in the nursing home, additional time is spent in contacting the prescriber, describing the situation, and deciding to go ahead with the stronger pain medicine. Because of the delay involved, patients in substantial pain are forced to leave the nursing home to go to the hospital where the process can take place more efficiently and pain relief can be rendered! The excess health care costs are, of course, in addition to the cost in pain and suffering.

While it is easy to place some blame on the changed policy in the DEA, those who created the state and federal laws that foster such an onerous climate must ultimately share the responsibility. Unfortunately, rarely are such individuals held accountable and good, vulnerable citizens suffer because of it.

A final suggestion on policy change has to do with an inherent problem within the justice system. Since older individuals have fewer years of anticipated survival and are less likely to have large amounts of potential damages, the more frail an individual, the less likely that any legal consequences will result from poor or even negligent care. Occasionally, there will be a sensational report, e.g., an award of $1.5 million before appeal in a landmark California lawsuit that invoked their elder abuse law [10]. This approach was necessary because, in California, the law does not allow collection of damages for pain and suffering after a patient has died. A few other spectacular awards have been seen as laws on this subject vary by state. For example, in 1990, a North Carolina jury awarded $15 million, before appeal, in damages against a nursing home where a nurse failed to administer prescribed pain medications to a terminally ill patient. In 1997, a South Carolina judge awarded $200,000 for undertreatment of a cancer patient's pain [11].

Because of variations in state laws, these cases are exceedingly rare, despite the prevalence of inadequate pain control among seniors. Without evidence of substantial damages and a high likelihood of a large settlement, an attorney will be very reluctant to take up a case involving a frail senior.

Communication

Whatever suggestions are made for changes to improve pain relief in the future, a high level of priority must be given to how pain issues are communicated. The news items such as noted above are helpful in spreading the message that inadequate pain management can have tangible consequences.

Communication efforts on pain relief must be augmented through the following:

- Health care systems
- Licensing boards
- Professional organizations
- Ethics committees
- Ombudsmen
- State surveyors
- Inspector General.

The public needs to hear about the lack of consistency within different health care systems, with regard to compliance and adherence to standards for pain management. Communication about access (or oftentimes lack thereof) is crucial. The message about the lack of research in pain management also needs to reach potential investigators as well as funding bodies. Communication about funding targeted toward such efforts is also vital to this effort.

To disseminate information on pain many resources must be used. Bringing government into collaboration with private organizations is a good start. The National Institute on Aging along with other NIH bodies has started to interact with not-for-profit entities. In part, this had been stimulated by reduced economic resources. This should be expanded. Partners would include such organizations as the American Cancer Society, the American Chronic Pain Association, and other nationally and internationally recognized organizations that focus on pain relief. Also local and statewide organizations should be identified to help promote a culturally sensitive educational media campaign to promote pain assessment and management. Communication within different health care systems regarding compliance and adherence to standards for pain management should also be a focus for positive and enlightened change.

The costs of communication will vary based on the media chosen. While public service announcements can be useful for television and radio, there is a tremendous demand on these venues. There will need to be strong governmental and administrative support to facilitate these types of efforts. The internet offers many potential avenues to explore for the distribution of information. Physician offices as well as the offices of other health care providers are wonderful resources for disseminating information. Brochures in such offices are often read, especially when there is an outdated magazine selection in the waiting room.

Churches and other places of spiritual worship should be recognized as wonderful places for dissemination of such information. Clergy should also be targets of communication and educational efforts because of the likelihood of their being approached for spiritual support during prolonged periods of pain (see Chap. 5).

Communicating via professional journals will be important because of the potential impact on centers of medical education. Efforts toward informing policy makers, including the politicians, are also worthwhile as long as there is a conscious evaluation of potential unintended consequences that may result due to implementation of additional policy changes, laws, and regulations.

It is also worth inviting the pharmaceutical industry and other portions of interested industry (medical devices, long-term care providers, durable medical equipment, etc.) to participate in promoting such efforts, recognizing the vested interest that exists. Such entities have great experience with communicating a message, i.e., marketing. Those working in the pain field would be wise to learn from those who understand marketing the best, from those who depend on being able to alter consumer behavior.

More on communication through the media is covered in Chaps. 11 and 13. Recommendations in dealing with the media are helpful for professionals as well. Regardless of the venue, being able to enunciate a concise, focused message will go a long way in advocating for those who continue to suffer with pain and to promote the laudable message of pain relief.

Conclusion

The opportunities for improving pain relief are many. Some are addressed in this chapter, e.g., improved educational efforts, research efforts, policy changes, and mechanisms for disseminating information. Others are addressed elsewhere throughout this book.

Pain does not discriminate. It can affect anyone regardless of race, creed, gender, political ideology, location, social status, or education. It can attack suddenly for short periods or last interminably. It can progress slowly and be persistent or wax and wane. Once it has served its brief educational purpose, it quickly becomes an unwelcome intruder. It can destroy lives and relationships. Pain starts with no bounds. Efforts and creativity to combat it must be boundless as well. Pain relief can be obtained. This book has offered practical advice to help achieve that relief for everyone suffering with pain. The message is an important one. We all must work to be sure that it is shared wherever the tentacles of pain might extend.

References

1. Ross JS, Hill KP, Egilman DS, Krumholz HM. Guest authorship and ghostwriting in publications related to rofecoxib: a case study of industry documents from rofecoxib litigation. JAMA. 2008;299:1800–12.
2. Ferrell BR, McGuire DM, Donovan MI. Knowledge and beliefs regarding pain in a sample of nursing faculty. J Prof Nurs. 1993;9(2):79–88.
3. Billings JA, Block JS. Palliative care in undergraduate medical education. Status report and future directions. JAMA. 1997;278(9):733–8.
4. Gloth FM. Credentialing, recertification, and public accountability. JAMA. 2006; 296:1587–8.
5. Zenz M, Willweber-Strumpf A. Opiophobia and cancer pain in Europe. Lancet. 1993; 341(8852):1075–6.
6. Keeler J. No More Paper. Advance for Health Information Executives. 2001; 51–4.
7. Drazen E, Killbridge P, Metzger J, Turisco F. A primer on physician order entry. Oakland, CA: California Healthcare Foundation; 2000. p. 1–44.
8. Centers for Medicare and Medicaid Services. http://www.medicare.gov/NHCompare/Search/Related/ImportantInformation.asp. Accessed 1 Feb 2003.
9. Maryland Health Care Commission. http://www.209.219.237.235/legal.htm. Accessed 1 Feb 2003.
10. Anonymous. Patient's family wins suit for undertreatment of pain. Prim Care Cancer. 2001;21:http://www.intouchlive.com/journals/primary/p0109h.htm
11. Anonymous. Pain management and the law. Am Assoc Phys Surg. 2001;57(8):3.

Index

CPSIA information can be obtained at www.ICGtesting.com
Printed in the USA
LVOW10*1803280414

383555LV00009B/304/P